HEALTH PROFESSIONS FACULTY FOR THE FUTURE

PROCEEDINGS OF A WORKSHOP

Patricia A. Cuff and Erin Hammers Forstag, *Rapporteurs*

Global Forum on Innovation in Health Professional Education

Board on Global Health

Health and Medicine Division

The National Academies of
SCIENCES · ENGINEERING · MEDICINE

THE NATIONAL ACADEMIES PRESS
Washington, DC
www.nap.edu

THE NATIONAL ACADEMIES PRESS 500 Fifth Street, NW Washington, DC 20001

This activity was supported by contracts between the National Academy of Sciences and Academic Collaborative for Integrative Health, Academy of Nutrition and Dietetics, Accreditation Council for Graduate Medical Education, Aetna Foundation, American Academy of Nursing, American Association of Colleges of Osteopathic Medicine, American Board of Family Medicine, American College of Obstetricians and Gynecologists, American Council of Academic Physical Therapy, American Dental Education Association, American Medical Association, American Nurses Credentialing Center, American Occupational Therapy Association, American Osteopathic Association, American Physical Therapy Association, American Psychological Association, American Speech-Language-Hearing Association, Association of American Medical Colleges, Association of American Veterinary Medical Colleges, Association of Schools and Colleges of Optometry, Association of Schools of Advancing Health Professions, Athletic Training Strategic Alliance, Council on Social Work Education, The George Washington University, Heron Therapeutics, Josiah Macy Jr. Foundation, Michigan Center for Interprofessional Education, National Academies of Practice, National Association of Social Workers, National Board for Certified Counselors and Affiliates, National Board of Medical Examiners, National Council of State Boards of Nursing, National League for Nursing, Physician Assistant Education Association, Society for Simulation in Healthcare, University of Toronto, U.S. Department of Veterans Affairs, and Weill Cornell Medicine–Qatar. Any opinions, findings, conclusions, or recommendations expressed in this publication do not necessarily reflect the views of any organization or agency that provided support for the project.

International Standard Book Number-13: 978-0-309-16011-7
International Standard Book Number-10: 0-309-16011-1
Digital Object Identifier: https://doi.org/10.17226/26041

Additional copies of this publication are available from the National Academies Press, 500 Fifth Street, NW, Keck 360, Washington, DC 20001; (800) 624-6242 or (202) 334-3313; http://www.nap.edu.

Copyright 2021 by the National Academy of Sciences. All rights reserved.

Printed in the United States of America

Cover credit: Front cover image created by John Hain, "Learning from Each Other."

Suggested citation: National Academies of Sciences, Engineering, and Medicine. 2021. *Health professions faculty for the future: Proceedings of a workshop*. Washington, DC: The National Academies Press. https://doi.org/10.17226/26041.

The National Academies of
SCIENCES · ENGINEERING · MEDICINE

The **National Academy of Sciences** was established in 1863 by an Act of Congress, signed by President Lincoln, as a private, nongovernmental institution to advise the nation on issues related to science and technology. Members are elected by their peers for outstanding contributions to research. Dr. Marcia McNutt is president.

The **National Academy of Engineering** was established in 1964 under the charter of the National Academy of Sciences to bring the practices of engineering to advising the nation. Members are elected by their peers for extraordinary contributions to engineering. Dr. John L. Anderson is president.

The **National Academy of Medicine** (formerly the Institute of Medicine) was established in 1970 under the charter of the National Academy of Sciences to advise the nation on medical and health issues. Members are elected by their peers for distinguished contributions to medicine and health. Dr. Victor J. Dzau is president.

The three Academies work together as the **National Academies of Sciences, Engineering, and Medicine** to provide independent, objective analysis and advice to the nation and conduct other activities to solve complex problems and inform public policy decisions. The National Academies also encourage education and research, recognize outstanding contributions to knowledge, and increase public understanding in matters of science, engineering, and medicine.

Learn more about the National Academies of Sciences, Engineering, and Medicine at **www.nationalacademies.org**.

The National Academies of
SCIENCES · ENGINEERING · MEDICINE

Consensus Study Reports published by the National Academies of Sciences, Engineering, and Medicine document the evidence-based consensus on the study's statement of task by an authoring committee of experts. Reports typically include findings, conclusions, and recommendations based on information gathered by the committee and the committee's deliberations. Each report has been subjected to a rigorous and independent peer-review process and it represents the position of the National Academies on the statement of task.

Proceedings published by the National Academies of Sciences, Engineering, and Medicine chronicle the presentations and discussions at a workshop, symposium, or other event convened by the National Academies. The statements and opinions contained in proceedings are those of the participants and are not endorsed by other participants, the planning committee, or the National Academies.

For information about other products and activities of the National Academies, please visit www.nationalacademies.org/about/whatwedo.

PLANNING COMMITTEE ON HEALTH PROFESSIONS FACULTY FOR THE FUTURE[1]

REAMER BUSHARDT (*Co-Chair*), The George Washington University
KATHY CHAPPELL (*Co-Chair*), American Nurses Credentialing Center
ANTHONY R. ARTINO, JR., The George Washington University School of Medicine and Health Sciences
SHELLEY COHEN KONRAD, University of New England
RODERIC I. PETTIGREW, Texas A&M University
NORMA IRIS POLL-HUNTER, Association of American Medical Colleges
LAWRENCE SHERMAN, Meducate Global, LLC

Consultants

KAREN PARDUE, University of New England
ALIKI THOMAS, McGill University

---

[1] The National Academies of Sciences, Engineering, and Medicine's planning committees are solely responsible for organizing the workshop, identifying topics, and choosing speakers. The responsibility for the published Proceedings of a Workshop rests with the rapporteurs and the institution.

Reviewers

This Proceedings of a Workshop was reviewed in draft form by individuals chosen for their diverse perspectives and technical expertise. The purpose of this independent review is to provide candid and critical comments that will assist the National Academies of Sciences, Engineering, and Medicine in making each published proceedings as sound as possible and to ensure that it meets the institutional standards for quality, objectivity, evidence, and responsiveness to the charge. The review comments and draft manuscript remain confidential to protect the integrity of the process.

We thank the following individuals for their review of this proceedings:

LISA HOWLEY, Association of American Medical Colleges
PHYLLIS M. KING, Association of Schools of the Allied Health Professions
JOANNE G. SCHWARTZBERG, Accreditation Council for Graduate Medical Education

Although the reviewers listed above provided many constructive comments and suggestions, they were not asked to endorse the content of the proceedings nor did they see the final draft before its release. The review of this proceedings was overseen by **PATRICK H. DeLEON,** Uniformed Services University of the Health Sciences. He was responsible for making certain that an independent examination of this proceedings was carried out in accordance with standards of the National Academies and that all review comments were carefully considered. Responsibility for the final content rests entirely with the rapporteurs and the National Academies.

Contents

1 INTRODUCTION 1

2 EVALUATING OUTCOMES BASED ON THOUGHTFUL
   PROGRAM DESIGNS (STEP 5) 7

3 BUILDING PATHWAYS AND BROADENING RECRUITMENT
   (STEPS 1 AND 2) 17

4 TRAINING NEW RECRUITS AND CURRENT FACULTY
   TO BE EFFECTIVE EDUCATORS (STEP 3) 27

5 BUILDING FACILITATING STRUCTURES FOR INFORMAL
   FACULTY DEVELOPMENT (STEP 4) 35

6 CLOSING REFLECTIONS 41

APPENDIXES
A MEMBERS OF THE GLOBAL FORUM ON INNOVATION
   IN HEALTH PROFESSIONAL EDUCATION 49
B WORKSHOP AGENDA 59
C SPEAKER BIOGRAPHICAL SKETCHES 63
D BEST ANDRAGOGICAL PRACTICES FOR ONLINE
   LEARNING AND FACULTY DEVELOPMENT 71
E FORUM-SPONSORED PRODUCTS 73

1

Introduction[1]

On August 11, 2020, the Global Forum on Innovation in Health Professional Education (the forum) held a virtual workshop titled Health Professions Faculty for the Future. The 3.5-hour workshop featured presentations from a variety of speakers and also used a chat box and live polling in order to encourage conversation among workshop participants.

The idea for the workshop, said Reamer Bushardt, senior associate dean in the School of Medicine and Health Sciences at The George Washington University and workshop committee member, originated from previous work of the forum. In November 2018, the forum jointly held a workshop with the National Center for Interprofessional Practice and Education called Strengthening the Connection Between Health Professions Education and Practice (NASEM, 2019). At that workshop, stakeholders from more than 15 different health professions came together from across the globe to present and discuss issues including education and training; patient-centered care; delivery and payment models; developing the workforce; and meeting the needs of populations, students, and educators. Workshop participants discussed the definition of a "health professions educator" and explored the knowledge, skills, and abilities that future health professions educators will need. A defining message of the workshop, said Bushardt, was that

---

[1] The planning committee's role was limited to planning the workshop, and this Proceedings of a Workshop was prepared by the rapporteurs as a factual account of what occurred at the workshop. Statements, recommendations, and opinions expressed are those of individual presenters and participants and are not necessarily endorsed or verified by the National Academies of Sciences, Engineering, and Medicine. They should not be construed as reflecting any group consensus.

partnership and alignment between education and practice is critical for success and is built on relationships. He also recollected how the workshop participants brainstormed about the barriers and opportunities for bridging the gap between education and practice, and they discussed the role health professions faculty would play in preparing the future workforce. The outcome was a vision for future health professions educators, said Bushardt, which laid the foundation for this workshop.

WHERE DID THE IDEA FOR HEALTH PROFESSIONS FACULTY FOR THE FUTURE ORIGINATE?

Reamer Bushardt, The George Washington University, and Kathy Chappell, American Nurses Credentialing Center

In preparation for this virtual workshop, Bushardt described his work with Kathy Chappell, senior vice president at the American Nurses Credentialing Center, in creating a pictorial image of a five-step framework for faculty development. Bushardt and Chappell developed their framework based on discussions and ideas generated from the 2018 joint workshop described previously, and they shared their thoughts with others on the workshop planning committee (see p. v). This framework—that aligns with the Statement of Task (see Box 1-1)—is a work in progress, said Bushardt. The workshop is an opportunity for participants to explore how this proposed framework might be tested, refined, and improved. It is hoped that the workshop's discussions will contribute to a common framework that can facilitate ongoing innovation in the health professions education community, he said. The ultimate goal is to build a health professions faculty for "shaping a workforce that can navigate a dynamic health care landscape, lead person and family-centered care, seamlessly integrate technology to improve health, and advance health equity."

Chappell emphasized the importance of thoughtful faculty development, noting that particularly in the era of coronavirus disease 2019 (COVID-19), faculty need the necessary knowledge and skills to be effective educators. She further remarked how there can sometimes be a tension between the role of *clinician* versus *teacher*, and that great clinicians who move into faculty positions are often not given the skills they need to be great teachers.

She then introduced the workshop participants to the framework that she and Bushardt developed (see Figure 1-1). There are other frameworks in the literature, noted Chappell, but after reviewing several of them, and realizing there are a fair number of overlapping elements, the two decided to tailor one that would be a better fit for this workshop.

The workshop emphasized diversity, equity, and inclusion—diversity of people and perspectives; equity in policy, practice, and position; and

BOX 1-1
Statement of Task

A planning committee of the National Academies of Sciences, Engineering, and Medicine will organize and convene a 1-day public workshop to explore various aspects of faculty development. Presentations will provide examples of how educators are using effective teaching strategies and of practices in health professional education. The workshop will emphasize the role of education in changing health systems that may include but are not limited to:

- Expanding educators' pedagogical and andragogical skills;
- Keeping up with content knowledge;
- Developing relationships across health professions and across sectors;
- Being aware of changes in health systems and being ready to adapt education as indicated;
- Learning, teaching, and applying new technologies and data-driven applications;
- Understanding faculty's role in assessing, mentoring, and providing constructive feedback to learners and colleagues; and
- Recognizing one's own limitations physically, mentally, and financially in order to minimize the negative effects of stress and prevent burnout.

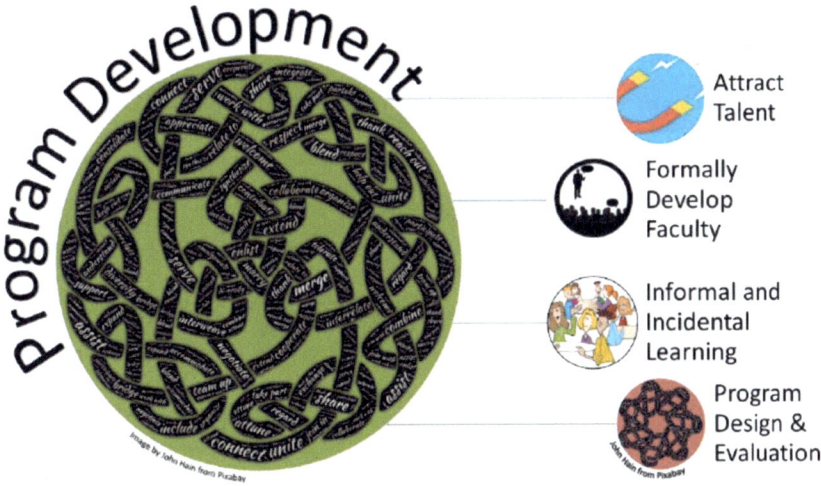

FIGURE 1-1 A framework for program development.
SOURCE: Presented by Bushardt and Chappell, August 11, 2020.

inclusion via power, voice, and organizational culture—within the four key areas shown in Figure 1-1. For this workshop, *diversity* is being defined broadly to include race, ethnicity, gender, sexual orientation, and people with physical disabilities, as well as diversity across health professions and sectors. Also of note, was the view that learning extends from education into practice, so the term *program development* (see Figure 1-1), was meant to include the educational spectrum from faculty development (in education) to continuing professional development (in practice). However, given the time limitations for the workshop, Chappell explained the speakers' primary focus was on faculty development.

Chappell encouraged workshop participants to give their feedback and input on the framework by using the chat box feature of the virtual meeting. She underscored the importance of participants' involvement as a critical review, including comments on what steps are missing, which steps work well and which need improvement, what enabling factors and barriers are anticipated, and whether the language used resonates with different health professions fields and stakeholders. "Workshop participants' input will be used to refine our framework," she said.

The organization of the workshop followed the five steps of the framework spelled out under four key areas (see Figure 1-2). Steps 1 and 2, building the pipeline and broadening recruitment into health professions education, both fall within the area of "attracting talent." Steps 3 through 5 work toward training faculty both formally and informally, and evaluating outcomes that are intricately linked to program design. However, Chappell

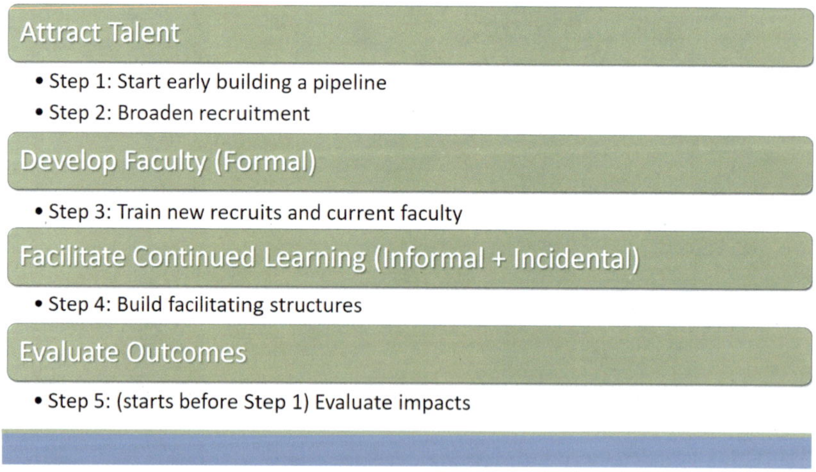

Attract Talent
- Step 1: Start early building a pipeline
- Step 2: Broaden recruitment

Develop Faculty (Formal)
- Step 3: Train new recruits and current faculty

Facilitate Continued Learning (Informal + Incidental)
- Step 4: Build facilitating structures

Evaluate Outcomes
- Step 5: (starts before Step 1) Evaluate impacts

FIGURE 1-2 A faculty development framework.
SOURCE: Presented by Bushardt and Chappell, August 11, 2020.

remarked, the workshop will "be starting with the end in mind," beginning with step 5. By identifying the goals and desired outcomes of a faculty development program first, said Chappell, this becomes the "north star" that guides the program and measures progress.

SETTING THE STAGE: WHAT WE LEARNED FROM YOU!

Lawrence Sherman, Meducate Global, LLC, and Association for Medical Education in Europe

Before diving into the framework, Lawrence Sherman, principal at Meducate Global, LLC, and international development expert at the Association for Medical Education in Europe (AMEE), shared some background on the planning of the workshop that aimed to bring out the interests of the participants expressed through a survey linked to registration. This survey, he said, provided an assessment of the "needs" of the 329 people who registered for the workshop. There were three main results from the responses expressing what registrants hoped to get out of attending the workshop (see Figure 1-3). First, registrants wanted as much interaction and engagement as possible, despite the virtual nature of the experience. Second, they wanted to see technology used to its full capacity. Sherman said this would be accomplished through the use of polls, chat boxes, and other interactive tools. Third, registrants wanted the workshop to serve as a model of best practices for virtual learning (see Appendix D). Sherman

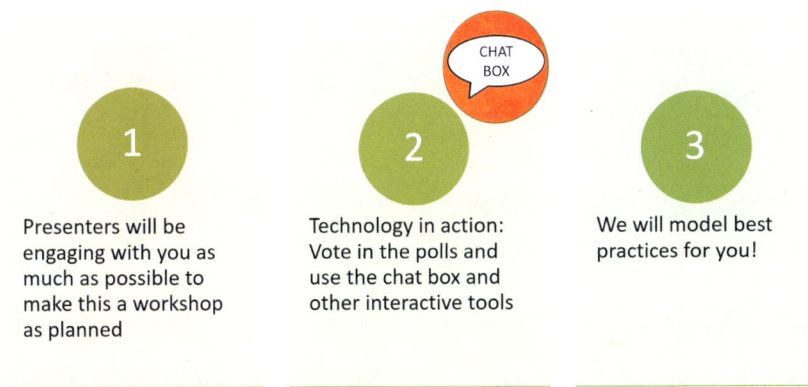

FIGURE 1-3 Attending to expressed needs and desires of workshop participants.
SOURCE: Presented by Sherman, August 11, 2020.

encouraged participants to give feedback in real time to be sure the workshop was meeting the needs and expectations of its attendees.

REFERENCE

NASEM (National Academies of Sciences, Engineering, and Medicine). 2019. *Strengthening the connection between health professions education and practice: Proceedings of a joint workshop*. Washington, DC: The National Academies Press. https://doi.org/10.17226/25407.

2

Evaluating Outcomes Based on Thoughtful Program Designs (Step 5)

HIGHLIGHTS[1]

- Faculty development is a knowledge translation activity. (Artino and Thomas)
- Using a framework can help guide the design, implementation, and evaluation of faculty development programs. (Thomas)
- There are limitations to using self-reported satisfaction surveys as evaluation tools. (Artino)

STARTING WITH THE END IN MIND: DESIGNING AND EVALUATING FACULTY DEVELOPMENT

Anthony Artino, The George Washington University, and Aliki Thomas, McGill University

Beginning with the end in mind, said Anthony Artino, tenured professor at The George Washington University, the fifth step of designing and evaluating faculty development becomes the first step. Faculty is defined broadly, said Artino, to include anyone who is involved with the education and training of health professionals, including professors, clinical teachers, and others. Artino's opening remarks drew comments in the chat box throughout

---

[1] This list at the beginning of each chapter is the rapporteurs' summary of the main points made by individual speakers (noted in parentheses). The statements have not been endorsed or verified by the National Academies of Sciences, Engineering, and Medicine. They are not intended to reflect a consensus among workshop participants.

the presentation and while he and Aliki Thomas, associate professor at McGill University, described a case example to illuminate their points (see Box 2-1) throughout the presentation, which was divided into three topics:

- Faculty development as a knowledge translation (KT) activity
- Using a framework to guide design
- Evaluation and sustainability

Faculty Development as a Knowledge Translation Activity

As part of best practices in virtual education, Thomas began by asking the workshop participants to complete the poll, "Is faculty development a knowledge translation intervention?" While many responded "yes," quite a few respondents indicated they were not sure what KT was. KT, said Thomas, is a process that aims to optimize the uptake of knowledge and scientific evidence to improve educational practices and policies (Thomas et al., 2014). Faculty development can be considered a KT activity because the goal is to increase or change the faculty's knowledge, skills, attitudes, and practices, with the ultimate goal of improving learner outcomes and eventually patient care. KT is divided into three steps, said Thomas (see Figure 2-1). The first step is identifying the research to practice (R-P) gap: what is the magnitude and nature of the gap between current practices and best practices in the literature? The second step is finding out why there is a gap: what are the factors that support or hinder the uptake of that

---

**BOX 2-1
Case Example**

You are a nurse practitioner in a large teaching hospital and have observed questionable feedback practices between staff (nurses and doctors) and students (and residents). Most recently, three students have complained to you that they do not receive timely feedback from their preceptors, that the feedback is frequently "hurtful," and that it does not focus on ways to improve. You would like to change and improve the ways in which feedback is provided in your center and are aware of the research on giving effective feedback. Your hope is that the teaching practices within your institution will be more aligned with those in the literature. Importantly, your ultimate goal is to make sure that learners can benefit from their experience and make good use of the feedback they receive so they may meet their learning goals.

SOURCE: Presented by Thomas, August 11, 2020.

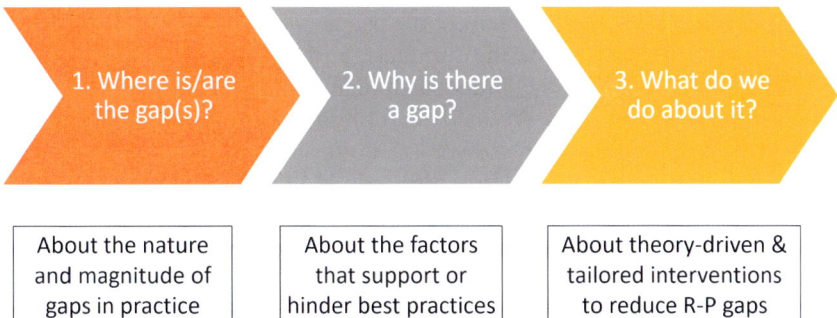

FIGURE 2-1 Three steps of knowledge translation.
SOURCES: Presented by Artino and Thomas, August 11, 2020. Data from Thomas and Bussières, 2016b.

evidence? Finally, the third step is determining what to do, using theory-driven and tailored interventions to reduce the gap.

In response to a workshop participant question, Thomas clarified that the term *knowledge translation* is an umbrella term. KT is a process used to address knowledge, skills, attitudes, behaviors, and other constructs, if they are the causes of the R-P gap, with the penultimate goal of promoting use of best practices. A gap between current practices and best practices might be due to a lack of knowledge, a lack of skills, or a specific attitude, she said. Once the reason for the gap is identified, the intervention would focus on making changes in that area. Thomas noted that in "knowledge translation" there are more than 100 different terms used to refer to the same process and that often terms such as *research use*, *diffusion*, *dissemination*, and *implementation* are used interchangeably although they mean different things. In the chat box, Warren Newton, president and chief executive officer for the American Board of Family Medicine, worried about knowledge being presented as binary or gaps, as opposed to higher-order "wisdom." Getting facts seems a low bar when compared to demonstrating implementation and critical skills. Artino agreed saying, "Education is about preparing participants for yet-to-be experienced problems." Sherman expounded on the idea suggesting faculty development be viewed as continuing professional development where there is ongoing assessment of the needs of the faculty, both as a group and as individuals.

Using a Framework to Guide Design

Changing behavior is a complex process, said Thomas, and faculty behavior takes place in complex clinical and educational environments. Using theories and frameworks can help to guide implementation efforts aimed at modifying behaviors. Implementation science is the scientific study of KT, said Thomas, and offers theories, models, and methods. Frameworks can help explain and predict the intended change and identify the multiple factors that can increase or decrease the likelihood that the change will occur. Furthermore, the use of a framework that considers different stakeholders emphasizes the notion that action plans should take into account the perspectives of all those who will be involved in and affected by the proposed change in behavior; such a framework also addresses issues of inclusion and diversity. There are multiple types of theories, models, and frameworks that can guide the design and evaluation of faculty development programs, including models that describe the process of translating research into practice, theories to explain what influences the outcomes, and frameworks to evaluate implementation.

Thomas presented a conceptual framework called the knowledge-to-action framework, which is based on a review of more than 30 planned-action theories (Graham et al., 2006) (see Figure 2-2). The knowledge-to-action framework takes local context and culture into account and offers a holistic

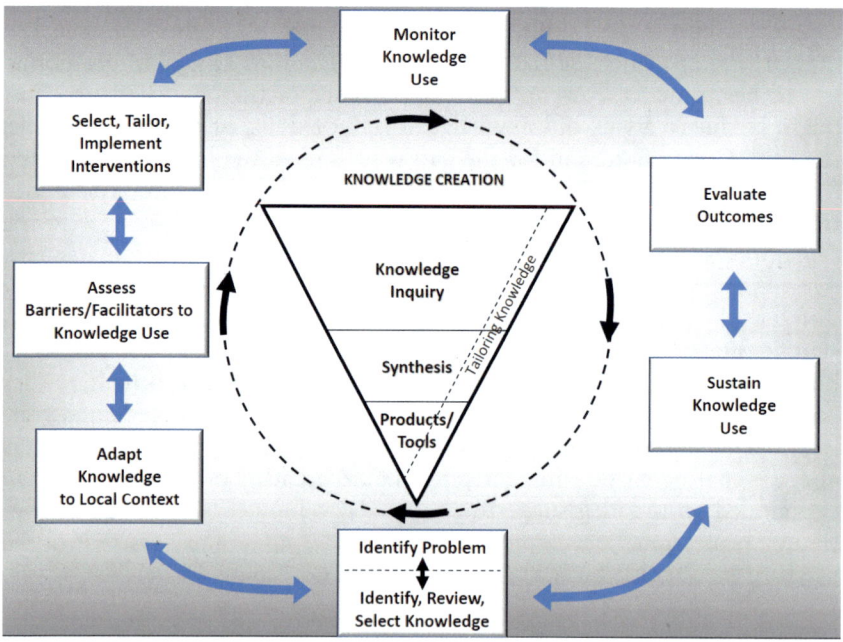

FIGURE 2-2 Knowledge-to-action framework.
SOURCES: Presented by Thomas, August 11, 2020. Data from Thomas and Bussières, 2016a.

view of the KT phenomenon. The framework considers how stakeholders will respond to anticipated changes and how change agents can facilitate the changes in educational practice. The funnel in the middle of the framework, said Thomas, represents the creation of knowledge from research findings and outcome evaluations that will be translated to the users. As the funnel becomes smaller, the knowledge becomes more synthesized and potentially more useful to the end users. The seven steps surrounding the funnel, while sequential in theory, might occur simultaneously, and there may be interactions between the steps as well as the knowledge base (e.g., if new evidence emerges). Thomas noted that the authors of the framework acknowledged that KT interventions rarely take place in environments where the knowledge gaps are clearly defined and where the actions required to change behavior are readily implementable and sustainable.

Looking at the framework with the aforementioned case example in mind (see Box 2-1), Thomas said the first step is identifying that the problem is "suboptimal feedback practices" in the teaching hospital. After identifying the problem, the literature is reviewed for evidence on strategies for giving effective feedback, and current feedback practices are examined in order to confirm the presence and nature of the gap between current practices and best practices. The second step is adapting the knowledge to the local context to ensure that it is relevant, applicable, and useful for the particular setting. At this step, said Thomas, it is critical to involve multiple stakeholders for their perspectives; in the case example, this could include teachers, learners, program directors, and curriculum chairs. The third step is assessing facilitators and barriers to knowledge use: what factors will make it more or less likely that feedback behavior will change? At this step, it is important to look at both individual and organizational facilitators and barriers (see Table 2-1).

TABLE 2-1 Some Individual and Organizational Facilitators and Barriers to Change

	Individual	Organizational
Facilitators	• Motivation to change • Readiness to change • Belief that feedback will result in better learner outcomes	• Protected time to read and discuss evidence on feedback • Proximity to university • Strong residency training
Barriers	• Heavy patient caseloads or lack of time to read literature • Lack of knowledge on effective feedback strategies • Lack of good role models	• Program with few resources to support uptake of new practices • No funds for faculty development • Lack of recognition of continuous professional development regarding educational issues

SOURCE: Presented by Thomas, August 11, 2020.

A workshop participant used the chat box to ask about systemic barriers; for example, faculty may have the knowledge about appropriate feedback but may have problems implementing it because of difficulty reconciling their dual roles of teacher and clinician. To mitigate these issues, it is critical to get a variety of stakeholders, including faculty, leaders, and managers, involved in the process "from the get-go," said Thomas. A participant shared her personal experience in the chat saying input from faculty is not widely sought for designing faculty development programs that truly address the needs of faculty. Bushardt responded, saying that this view "is not all that different from patients' involvement (or lack thereof) across health care delivery, [but] that's hopefully changing now with more focus on person-centered care paradigms."

The fourth step is selecting, tailoring, and implementing the actual KT intervention, Thomas explained. At this step, the faculty development activity (as the KT intervention) is implemented to try to reduce the gap between current practices and best practices. For example, if the gap is a lack of knowledge on how to give effective feedback, the intervention could be giving faculty regularly scheduled, online opportunities to learn and to practice feedback. This step includes (1) considering who needs to do what differently and how, (2) the involvement of multiple stakeholders to promote uptake of new strategies, and (3) an examination of KT interventions in the literature. Thomas noted, in response to a participant's question, that interventions should be chosen based on whether evidence in the literature supports use of the intervention. After the intervention is implemented, the fifth step is monitoring knowledge use. This could include looking for measurable changes in knowledge, attitudes, skills, and behaviors, such as increased knowledge about effective feedback or improved feedback practices.

Evaluation and Sustainability

The sixth step of the knowledge-to-action framework—and an essential part of any faculty development program—is evaluation. Artino defined evaluation as the "systematic acquisition and assessment of information to provide useful feedback about some object" (Trochim, 2006), and its goal is to "determine the merit or worth of some thing" (Cook, 2010). In the case of faculty development, the "object" or the "thing" being evaluated is the faculty development program. There are three reasons that one might conduct an evaluation, said Artino. The first is to be accountable for the time, money, and effort that have been invested in the faculty development program. The second is to generate understandings and new insights about what is working and what is not working. The third reason is to support and guide improvement of the faculty development program.

Evaluation is both similar to and different from research, said Artino. Research is broader, and is often aimed at discovering generalizable knowledge, understanding, or theory. However, many of the same precepts apply to both evaluation and research: both should ask relevant questions, be rigorous, use appropriate methods, adhere to ethical principles, and report and disseminate findings. Artino noted that dissemination does not have to be national or international; local dissemination to key stakeholders is relevant and important. One key difference between evaluation and research, said Artino, is that evaluation is often situated in a "potentially sensitive political and ethical context" with many different stakeholders, including policy makers, funders, regulators, teachers, and students. When considering evaluation, it is helpful to consider the different perspectives and goals of these stakeholders, he said.

Even after evaluation of a faculty development program, said Thomas, there is one more step. It is essential to ensure the sustainability of knowledge; that is, to ensure that the changes in knowledge or behavior last past the "honeymoon period" of a month or two. One strategy for sustainability is having a "champion" on site, who can hold regular meetings with the team, have regular check-ins with team members, and ensures that the program remains a priority.

What and How to Evaluate

Evaluation is often framed as a way to answer the question "Does the faculty development program work?" However, said Artino, framing it in this way suggests a quasi-experimental design that looks for a clear, linear relationship between the program and changes in attitudes, learning, and behavior. Instead, he said, it may be more helpful to consider the question, "Why does the faculty development program work (or not), for whom, and under what circumstances?" While this framing is more complex and requires evaluating multiple constructs, it invites a nuanced, mixed methods, holistic approach to evaluation. A program evaluation might look at both proximal and distal constructs, said Thomas. A proximal construct would be, for example, changes in the feedback practices of a particular teacher. A distal construct could be the knowledge of the learner, and ultimately his or her performance as a health care professional. This type of construct, while more important in the long run, is more difficult to measure. To select relevant and feasible constructs for evaluation, said Thomas, it is essential to have multiple stakeholders at the table to lend their perspectives.

In the case example, said Thomas, one could measure outcomes such as the number of learners receiving appropriate feedback, the nature and frequency of feedback, or teachers' and students' self-reported experience of the feedback interaction. Measuring these types of outcomes can be done with a variety of methods (see Table 2-2). Surveys and questionnaires are common ways to measure knowledge, attitudes, practices, and self-efficacy, while observation can be an effective way to measure actual practice and competence. Ideally, said Artino, multiple evaluation methods would be combined to gather the most robust evidence about outcomes. One method that is frequently used for evaluation is the "butts-in-seats" measure, which simply reports the number of people trained or educated. This measure, Artino said, is like "evaluating how you did in a battle by how many bullets you used." The number of program participants is a useful starting point but cannot be the end of the evaluation.

Using Surveys for Evaluation

A method that is frequently used to evaluate faculty development or other educational programs is a self-reported survey of satisfaction, also called a "smile sheet," said Artino. Workshop participants were polled on whether smile sheets are a good way to collect outcome data for evaluation purposes; while many said yes, more replied no. Artino said that the literature on this issue is a bit "all over the map," but that the most recent literature suggests that satisfaction surveys are a poor way to evaluate learning outcomes. A recent meta-analysis (Uttl et al., 2017) looked at 51 published studies on satisfaction surveys, and found that satisfaction ratings are "essentially unrelated to learning." In other words, said Artino, being satisfied with the course is usually unrelated to how much was learned in the course.

Another study found that providing participants with cookies at the end of a course session could create statistically significant and very large increases in the ratings of the course, course materials, and teachers (Hessler et al., 2018). In addition, satisfaction surveys have been shown to be biased against a number of groups, including women, minorities, and short people,

TABLE 2-2 Examples of Various Methods for Measuring Outcomes

Construct	Method
Knowledge	Survey, vignette, test
Attitudes	Survey, standardized questionnaire, interviews
Self-reported practices	Survey, standardized questionnaire, interviews
Self-efficacy	Survey, standardized questionnaire, interviews
Actual practice	Observation, chart audit, video recall
Competence	Simulation, vignettes, observation, videoconference

SOURCE: Presented by Artino, August 11, 2020.

said Artino. A workshop participant asked how to mitigate this type of bias, and Artino responded that even with a high-quality, well-written satisfaction survey, bias will likely still exist. He encouraged people to focus on measuring the specific skills, knowledge, and behaviors that the activity is designed to change, rather than measuring satisfaction with the course or the instructor.

The crucial message, said Artino, is that smile sheets are of limited value, and rigorous evaluation of faculty development needs to use other methods. However, he said, surveys can still provide valuable evaluation data if they are well designed, linked to theory or a framework, and focused on constructs beyond satisfaction. For example, surveys can be used to measure outcomes such as self-reported knowledge, attitudes, or practice patterns. He noted that the literature is replete with examples of validated surveys that measure these types of constructs, so there is no need to "reinvent the wheel." Even when validated, surveys should be reviewed with an eye toward how they will function in the particular setting and population, and they should always be pretested before using.

REFERENCES

Cook, D. A. 2010. Twelve tips for evaluating educational programs. *Medical Teacher* 32(4):296–301. doi: 10.3109/01421590903480121.

Graham, I. D., J. Logan, M. B. Harrison, S. E. Straus, J. Tetroe, W. Caswell, and N. Robinson. 2006. Lost in knowledge translation: Time for a map? *Journal of Continuing Education for Health Professionals* 26:13–24.

Hessler, M., D. M. Pöpping, H. Hollstein, H. Ohlenburg, P. H. Arnemann, C. Massoth, L. M. Seidel, A. Zarbock, and M. Wenk. 2018. Availability of cookies during an academic course session affects evaluation of teaching. *Medical Education* 52:1064–1072.

Thomas, A., and A. Bussières. 2016a. Knowledge translation and implementation science in health professions education: Time for clarity? *Academic Medicine* 91(12):e20. https://doi.org/10.1097/ACM.0000000000001396.

Thomas, A., and A. Bussières. 2016b. Towards a greater understanding of implementation science in health professions education. *Academic Medicine* 91(12):e19. https://doi.org/10.1097/ACM.0000000000001441.

Thomas, A., A. Menon, J. Boruff, A. M. Rodriguez, and S. Ahmed. 2014. Applications of social constructivist learning theories in knowledge translation for healthcare professionals: A scoping review. *Implementation Science* 9:54. https://doi.org/10.1186/1748-5908-9-54.

Trochim, W. M. K. 2006. *Evaluation research.* http://www.socialresearchmethods.net/kb/evaluation.php (accessed December 15, 2020).

Uttl, B., C. White, and D. Gonzalez. 2017. Meta-analysis of faculty's teaching effectiveness: Student evaluation of teaching ratings and student learning are not related. *Studies in Educational Evaluation* 54:22–24.

3

Building Pathways and Broadening Recruitment (Steps 1 and 2)

HIGHLIGHTS

- Building diverse faculty members begins long before health professions school. (Sánchez)
- Formal pre-faculty development can help recruit, retain, and support diverse practitioners and faculty. (Sánchez)
- There are multiple factors that facilitate or inhibit a person's decision to pursue a faculty career, including visibility and representation of diverse faculty. (Sánchez)
- It is a professional obligation for faculty to pull others "up the ladder." (Chappell)

Kathy Chappell introduced the moderator and speaker of the next session, Norma Poll-Hunter, senior director at the Association of American Medical Colleges, and John Paul Sánchez, director of the learning environment fellowship from the University of New Mexico, whose personal and professional experiences guided the participants through steps 1 and 2 of the framework. To begin, said Chappell, the title selected for these steps looks to build an early "pipeline" into health professions education, but it was brought to the attention of the planning committee while preparing for the workshop that a pipeline can be seen as a straight line into the health professions. This may not be indicative of how many from underserved communities find their way into the health professions, which may more resemble a series of "on" and "off-ramps" in career development. This speaks to the fluidity of the framework where building pathways (versus a pipeline) into education and broadening recruitment—particularly with a lens of diversity, equity, and inclusion—will be incorporated.

PRE-FACULTY DEVELOPMENT: A CRITICAL FACTOR IN DIVERSIFYING HEALTH PROFESSIONS FACULTY

John Paul Sánchez, Health Sciences Center, University of New Mexico

Pre-faculty development is a critical factor in diversifying health professions faculty, said Sánchez, who is also president and founder of Building the Next Generation of Academic Physicians (BNGAP). Building a diverse and inclusive next generation of faculty requires starting early by broadening recruitment and building a pathway to health professions education. There are a number of significant challenges in diversifying health professions faculty, said Sánchez; however, there are also numerous opportunities to engage with students and prepare them to become the faculty of the future.

Sánchez began by reflecting on his own journey to becoming a faculty member. Sánchez is of Puerto Rican ancestry and grew up in the Bronx, New York. During college, Sánchez participated in formal programs that strengthened his academic skills and awareness of professional opportunities, gave him reassurance that he would be valued in becoming a practitioner, and helped him develop a professional portfolio. As a person of color, said Sánchez, these formal programs helped him in attaining his master in public health and his medical degree. Sánchez asked the other workshop participants to reflect on their own journeys and to share in the chat box responses to "When did you first gain formal guidance on becoming an educator or faculty member?" A selection of responses is shown in Box 3-1. Sánchez noted that many of his colleagues and mentors had little formal guidance on the way to becoming faculty members, and that they tend to report the rise to faculty as "serendipitous," "happenstance," or "incidental."

When considering why health professional education has not achieved greater diversity within the faculty workforce, said Sánchez, it is important to reflect on the lack of diversity even within the practitioner workforce. A significant factor in building a diverse faculty is for diverse individuals to first be practitioners, he said. As seen in Tables 3-1 and 3-2, African Americans, Hispanics, and American Indians together make up about 30 percent of the U.S. population; however, the proportion of graduate students, practitioners, and faculty from these groups is significantly lower than 30 percent. Within specific health professions, the disparity is even greater; for example, Hispanics make up around 16 percent of the U.S. workforce, but only 3.7 percent of pharmacists and chiropractors are Hispanic (HRSA, 2017).

> **BOX 3-1**
> **Key Points Made by Individual Participants**
>
> Sánchez asked participants to reflect on the opportunities that helped them become educators and/or faculty members. Here are some responses:
>
> - I received a master's in nursing education. (Regina Beard)
> - In my doctoral program, and it was choice, not required. (Shelley Cohen Konrad)
> - As a student tutor at the Medical University of South Carolina, the director at the Center for Academic Excellence developed us as "supplemental instructors" versus tutors. Training blended with lots of encouragement, safe practice, and feedback. (Reamer Bushardt)
> - I never had formal guidance. My mother was a part-time and full-time faculty member at Emory University. (Christine Wright)
> - It wasn't until I asked someone about it that someone gave me some direction. I was already a practicing clinician. (Lori Bordenave)
> - During physician assistant (PA) school, advisors encouraged me to consider education due to my thesis and participation in interprofessional activities. (Shani Fleming)
> - When I was an undergraduate, one of my professors, an Ed.D., encouraged me to teach with him, and I was hooked! (Lawrence Sherman)
> - A faculty member took an interest in me and my career. (Valarie Fleming)
> - All of my guidance was informal. I came into the field of PA education as a medical technologist and crafted my own journey with informal responses from established faculty! (Janie McDaniel)
> - I did not receive formal guidance when considering transition from clinical work to academia. Honestly, was ill prepared for the experience … since then have unofficial mentors I use … one of whom is on this webinar. (Lydia Navarro-Walker)
> - My "formal training" was only mentorship from the only other faculty member at our very small program. It continues to this day; more of a give-and-take now that I feel like I have something to offer. (Kevin)
>
> SOURCE: Adapted from the presentation by Sánchez, August 11, 2020.

Sánchez said there are two significant disparities that need attention: one, representation within practitioner ranks, and two, representation within faculty ranks. Faculty are critical in many ways, said Sánchez, because they serve as role models and mentors to students and new professionals, they are champions for programs and policies, and they sit on admissions and other important committees. Sánchez asked "What factors influence an individual's trajectory to a faculty career, particularly diverse individuals?" Poll-Hunter, who works within AAMC's Diversity Policy and Programs unit, quickly scanned the responses for the most common

TABLE 3-1 U.S. Health Occupations by Race/Ethnicity, 2011–2015

	Hispanic	White
U.S. Workforce[a] (#)	25,776,728	102,850,895
U.S. Workforce[a] (%)	16.1	64.4
Health Occupations[b] (%)		
Community and Social Services Occupations		
Counselors	10.7	64.6
Social Workers	12.0	60.6
Life, Physical, and Social Sciences Occupations		
Psychologists	6.3	83.5
Health Diagnosing and Treating Practitioners Occupations		
Advanced Practice Registered Nurses[c]	4.5	84.0
Chiropractors	3.7	86.7
Dentists	6.1	74.8
Dietitians and Nutritionists	8.5	68.7
Optometrists	3.9	78.4
Pharmacists	3.7	70.4
Physicians	6.3	67.0
Physician Assistants	10.0	72.7
Occupational Therapists	4.0	83.8
Physical Therapists	4.8	77.8

[a] Population 16 years and older who are employed or seeking employment.
[b] Self-reported occupations.
[c] Includes nurse anesthetists, midwives, and nurse practitioners.
NOTES: Occupations are titled and grouped as in the U.S. government's Standard Occupation Classification system. NR = data not reported because relative standard errors (RSE) > 30; estimate does not meet standards of reliability or data not present. Numbers in parenthesis represent estimates with relative standard errors (RSE) > 20 percent and should be interpreted with caution. Not all totals equal to 100 percent due to rounding.
SOURCES: Presented by Sánchez, August 11, 2020; HRSA Sex, Race, and Ethnic Diversity of U.S. Health Occupations (2011–2015) 2017 Report.

	Non-Hispanic				
Black	Asian	American Indian/Alaska Native	Native Hawaiian and Other Pacific Islander	Multiple/Other Race
---	---	---	---	---
18,597,223	8,534,837	902,977	251,578	2,910,645
11.6	5.3	0.6	0.2	1.8
18.8	2.8	0.8	0.1	2.2
21.5	3.0	0.8	0.1	2.0
4.9	3.4	0.2	(0.0)	1.6
5.7	4.1	0.2	NR	1.3
1.9	5.4	0.5	NR	1.8
3.0	14.3	(0.1)	NR	1.7
15.0	6.0	0.3	(0.1)	1.4
1.8	13.7	NR	NR	1.8
5.9	17.9	0.2	0.1	1.8
4.8	19.6	0.1	0.0	2.1
7.1	7.3	0.6	NR	2.2
4.4	6.6	0.2	NR	1.1
4.4	11.1	0.2	(0.1)	1.6

TABLE 3-2 Approximate Hispanic, African American/Black, and American Indian/Alaska Native Population and U.S. Workforce Demographics by Discipline, 2015

	Population %	Graduate Students %	Clinicians %	Faculty %
Physician Assistant	30	10	11	10
Medicine	30	15	10	7
Dentist	30	12	7	15

NOTE: American Indian or Alaska Native plus Native Hawaiian and Other Pacific Islanders for data of census, graduates, and faculty.
SOURCES: Presented by Sánchez, August 11, 2020; AAMC, 2020; NCCPA, 2020; U.S. Census Bureau, 2020.

themes, which included mentorship, sponsors, seeing diverse faculty as role models, academic advisors, and leadership (see Box 3-2). These responses highlighted the importance of the role of others in either identifying or inspiring individuals to pursue faculty careers.

Given the responses of the workshop participants, Sánchez noted that "the problem is definitely multifactorial." He shared two frameworks to help elucidate the various factors that contribute to recruitment, retention, and success of faculty. The first was an adaptation of a framework on social determinants of health (see Figures 3-1a and 3-1b), which Sánchez called "determinants of health in academia." The second framework was a modified model of social cognitive career theory, and it includes factors that influence a person's career decision making (see Figure 3-2). Sánchez shared anonymous quotes from three potential faculty members that illuminate some of the factors that may prevent diverse students from considering faculty careers:

- Self-doubt about being good enough: "I don't know that my grades are as stellar as they should be because I picture an academic teacher

---

BOX 3-2
Key Points Made by Individual Participants

Sánchez asked workshop participants to reflect on what factors they believe influence an individual's trajectory to a faculty career. These are some results:

- Mentors with whom I identify. (Miguel Paniagua)
- Seeing someone from your diverse group as a faculty. (Christine Wright)
- Role models, financial aid for education, lower barriers for entry. (Peter Cahn)
- Personal connection, alignment with personal mission, mentorship. (Shani Fleming)
- Encouragement from senior faculty; good teaching in the classroom as role models. (Janelle O'Connell)
- Encouragement and role models. (Virginia Valentin)
- Visibility, representation. (Emelia)
- Factors include good role models, identifying potential learners who show promise as a future educator. (Melanie Bowzer)
- Leadership, leadership, leadership. (Holly Humphrey)
- Early exposure to mentors! Exposure to career fields within health care is another major influence. (Alice Vestergaard)
- Seeing and knowing people that look like me involved in the positions. (Lemmietta McNeilly)

SOURCE: Adapted from the presentation by Sánchez, August 11, 2020.

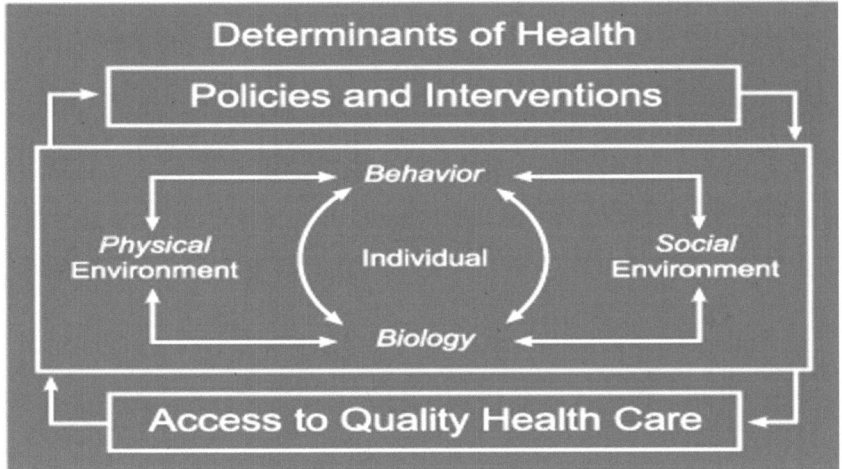

FIGURE 3-1a Original determinants of health framework.
SOURCES: Presented by Sánchez, August 11, 2020; adapted from Satcher and Higginbotham, 2008.

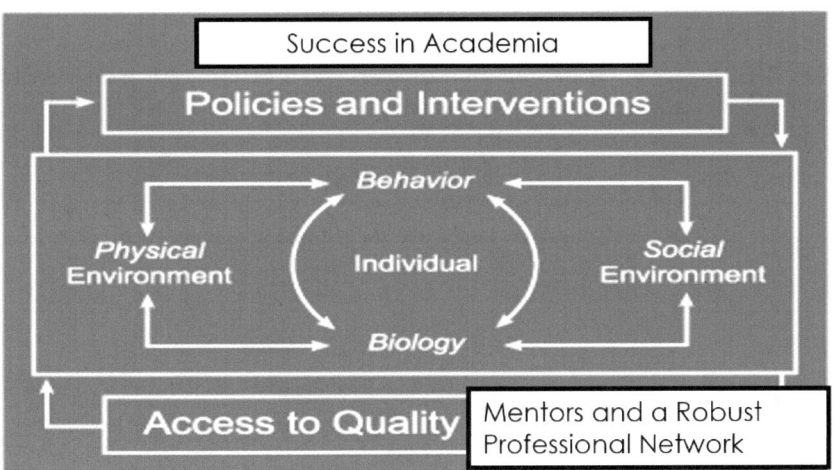

FIGURE 3-1b Adapted determinants of health and determinants of success in the academia framework.
SOURCES: Presented by Sánchez, August 11, 2020; adapted from Satcher and Higginbotham, 2008.

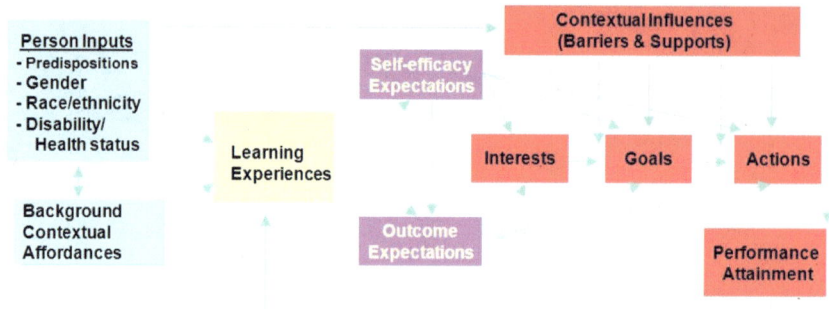

FIGURE 3-2 Modified model of social cognitive career theory.
SOURCES: Presented by Sánchez, August 11, 2020; adapted from Lent et al., 1994.

as somebody with excellent grades and I'm just kind of a floater. I'm not really someone who stands out academically. I mean, obviously we all stand out as medical students, but among those I'm pretty average. I would love to do it, but I don't think I have the research or the academic excellence" (Sanchez et al., 2013).
- Parents' view of clinical versus faculty careers: "I think a lot of people in our parents' generation, especially among Asian immigrants, see clinical practice as the 'iron rice bowl.' Basically, once you get the training, you can keep on eating out of it with a steady income and steady job" (Zhang et al., 2017).
- Difficulty finding LGBT mentors: "I haven't had any mentors, and I feel like because I lack that, I kind of want to provide support later on. There are no mentors who do research or teaching in LGBT health or who are out or who are supporting or very supportive of people who might be out in academic medicine" (Sanchez et al., 2015).

Sánchez then stated:

If we're serious about diversifying our faculty workforce, if we're serious about creating equitable processes in the recruitment, retention, and promotion of our faculty, and if we're serious about creating a sense of belonging, attention must be paid to pre-faculty development.

Sánchez defined pre-faculty development as providing potential faculty with "foundational self-efficacy, knowledge, skills, and experiences to be successfully appointed, and eventually promoted and tenured, within an academic institution" (Sánchez and Williams, 2020). Sánchez asked workshop participants to reflect on what types of formal pre-faculty development programs were a part of their journey. Poll-Hunter scanned the responses in the chat box and noted that the common theme among them was there are "not a lot of resources for pre-faculty development." Sánchez agreed with this assessment, and said that he never had formal pre-faculty development, despite having served in various faculty positions and as a dean. As a consequence, it is extremely gratifying for Sánchez to help his trainees and to give them a better experience than he had.

Sánchez told participants about his organization—Building the Next Generation of Academic Physicians (BNGAP, 2020)—that is aimed at supporting pre-faculty development. The mission of BNGAP is to "help diverse trainees become aware of, interested in, and prepared to explore academic careers." The group started by engaging with diverse trainees to understand the perceived challenges and facilitators to becoming future faculty, said Sánchez. The information that was gathered served to develop educational interventions to support a diverse pre-faculty workforce and to help build a pre-faculty identity for trainees. At each step of the way, the organization assesses outcomes and effects. BNGAP originally focused on medicine, but it has been adapted for dentistry, nursing, pharmacy, and public health.

Three concepts have emerged through the work of BNGAP, Sánchez said. First, it is critical to build community through conferences, chapters, newsletters, and by identifying role models and mentors who can connect with pre-faculty to keep them on track. One community-building entity, said Sánchez, is the BNGAP National Center for Pre-Faculty Development, which is a resource for networking and sharing best practices. Second, BNGAP seeks to address and dispel misconceptions about being a diverse faculty member. One example is the "minority tax" (extra responsibilities placed on minority faculty in the name of diversity);[1] BNGAP encourages trainees to transform this "tax" into "capital" by seeking writing fellowships or publishing opportunities. Finally, BNGAP helps trainees build career knowledge and skills through curricula that have been developed. There are curricula aimed at a variety of audiences ranging from college students to graduate students to those finding their first faculty position. Sánchez added that it is not only critical to encourage trainees to become faculty, but also to become deans and chairs of departments.

In closing, Sánchez encouraged workshop participants to take three steps after the workshop. First, keep talking about pre-faculty development, with colleagues, leaders, and trainees. Second, he encouraged collaboration to build formal, interprofessional pathway programs for a diverse pre-faculty. Third, he asked participants to "turn to a diverse trainee" and tell

---

[1] See https://bmcmededuc.biomedcentral.com/articles/10.1186/s12909-015-0290-9 (accessed December 9, 2020).

them, "I want you to be a future faculty member. I am here to answer any questions that you may have, and I'm going to tell you how great it is to be a faculty member." Sánchez encouraged participants to reach out to trainees to make them aware of potential faculty careers, to cultivate their interest in education, and to recognize the work they already do as educators. This type of conversation, said Sánchez, was fundamental for his journey, and it "does not require funding or protected time, and it is something really easy that we can all do." Chappell agreed with Sánchez, and added that at a certain point in a professional's career, it is a "professional obligation to reach back and pull somebody up the ladder."

REFERENCES

AAMC (Association of American Medical Colleges). 2020. *Medical education facts: Applicants, matriculants, enrollment, graduates, MD-PhD, and residency applicants data.* https://www.aamc.org/data-reports/students-residents/report/facts (accessed December 15, 2020).

BNGAP (Building the Next Generation of Academic Physicians). 2020. *About BNGAP.* http://bngap.org/about-us (accessed December 15, 2020).

HRSA (Health Resources and Services Administration). 2017. *HRSA Sex, Race, and Ethnic Diversity of U.S. Health Occupations (2011–2015) 2017 Report.* https://bhw.hrsa.gov/sites/default/files/bureau-health-workforce/data-research/diversity-us-health-occupations.pdf (accessed December 15, 2020).

Lent, R. W., S. D. Brown, and G. Hackett. 1994. Toward a unifying social cognitive theory of career and academic interest, choice, and performance. *Journal of Vocational Behavior* 45(1):79–122.

NCCPA (National Commission on Certification of Physician Assistants). 2020. *Reports.* https://www.nccpa.net/news-press.aspx?id=63&page=1&category=2&newsPressYear=2020 (accessed December 15, 2020).

Sánchez, J. P., and V. N. Williams. 2020. Introduction. In *Succeeding in academic medicine: A roadmap for diverse medical students and residents,* edited by J. P. Sánchez. Cham, Switzerland: Springer Nature. P. viii. https://doi.org/10.1007/978-3-030-33267-9.

Sánchez, J. P., L. Peters, E. Lee-Rey, H. Strelnick, G. Garrison, K. Zhang, D. Spencer, G. Ortega, B. Yehia, A. Berlin, and L. Castillo-Page. 2013. Racial and ethnic minority medical students' perceptions of academic medicine careers. *Academic Medicine* 88(9):1299–1307.

Sánchez, N., S. Rankin, E. Callahan, H. Ng, L. Holaday, K. McIntosh, N. Poll-Hunter, and J. P. Sánchez. 2015. LGBT health professionals perspectives on academic careers—Facilitators and challenges. *LGBT Health* 2(4):346–357. https://pdfs.semanticscholar.org/5aa5/b29ff7a4c387ffd782147f302c55bc8d373a.pdf (accessed December 15, 2020).

Satcher, D., and E. J. Higginbotham. 2008. The public health approach to eliminating disparities in health. *American Journal of Public Health* 98(9 Suppl):S8–S11.

U.S. Census Bureau. 2020. *Explore data.* https://www.census.gov/data.html (accessed December 15, 2020).

Zhang, L., Lee, E. S., Kenworthy, C. A., Chiang, S., Holaday, L., Spencer, D. J., Poll-Hunter, N. I., & Sánchez, J. P. 2017. Asian medical students' perceptions of careers in medicine. *Journal of Career Development* 46(3):235–250. https://doi.org/10.1177/0894845317740225 (accessed December 27, 2020).

4

Training New Recruits and Current Faculty to Be Effective Educators (Step 3)

HIGHLIGHTS

- The content, context, and methods used in education are never neutral, and there are always power dynamics at play. (Cohen Konrad)
- Instructors have a responsibility to create an environment where learners feel safe to make mistakes, propose alternative views, and have honest discussion. (Cohen Konrad)
- Using a framework for education can encourage self-awareness, restoration, and growth. (Pardue)

CONSCIOUS INSTRUCTION: AWARENESS, RESTORATION, AND GROWTH IN KNOWLEDGE TRANSFER

Shelley Cohen Konrad, Karen Pardue, and Kris Hall, University of New England

The third step of faculty development, said Shelley Cohen Konrad, director of the University of New England's (UNE's) Center for Excellence in Collaborative Education (CECE), is formal education or training that takes places in the classroom or workplace. Cohen Konrad, along with her colleagues from UNE, Karen Pardue, dean of Westbrook College of Health Professions, and Kris Hall, program manager of CECE, developed a framework called "conscious instruction." This framework, said Cohen

Konrad, calls attention to the "what, how, and why of education" and the choices that are made in every aspect of knowledge transfer.

Before presenting the framework, Pardue introduced workshop participants to some key terms used in their presentation (see Box 4-1), and Hall asked participants to reflect on the type of educator that they aspire to be. Responses, submitted through a computer polling app, included

- Engaging
- Humble
- Impactful
- Role model
- Innovative
- Norm shattering
- Connected to practice
- Quietly influencing

To explore the different dimensions of the conscious instruction framework, Cohen Konrad showed participants a video case study, which was created by an interprofessional team for students at UNE. The video

---

BOX 4-1
Key Terms

Courageous conversations, critical conversations, and brave conversations: Conversations that seek honest dialogue primarily aimed at understanding and discussing race, difference, discrimination, and systemic racism (Brown, 2018).

Knowledge transfer: The intentional process of imparting information as applied to subject content and associated skills within a learning context. The term is synonymous with *knowledge translation*. Knowledge transfer and translation are contextual, influenced by instruction, evidence, institutional culture, and implicit biases.

Psychological safety: The belief that one can express their views and perspectives without fear of negative repercussions. Learning environments must establish psychological safety before honest dialogue can ensue (Edmondson, 1999).

Radical listening: Being curious about what is being said and getting back to the speaker resisting the desire to tell your story, offer your opinion, or offer solutions (Tobin, 2009).

SOURCE: Presented by Cohen Konrad, August 11, 2020.

> **BOX 4-2**
> **Transcript Video Case Study**
>
> Pat Chalmers is a 31-year-old woman who prides herself in self-sufficiency and resourcefulness. She works part-time as a bookkeeper and takes care of her aging grandmother with whom she lives. Pat describes herself as having been a caretaker since adolescence. It is therefore difficult for her to acknowledge her own needs or to seek help from others. Pat is tired of people commenting on her weight, diet, and need to exercise. She avoids health care as much as possible because she knows she'll be told to lose weight or be blamed for being fat, in her words. "I know what risks I face," she says, "but I've tried everything, and nothing works. I can accept myself for the way I am, and I don't understand how others can't accept me for who I am. It's none of their business, really."
>
> Although her dental hygienist has urged her to seek out a primary care physician, Pat does not have a primary care physician when she finds herself in the emergency department with an ankle broken significantly enough to require surgery. Labs reveal elevated glucose levels, indicating possible type 2 diabetes, and surgery is postponed until further tests can be done to determine whether Pat might have diabetes. When asked about this possibility Pat reacts strongly: "I don't have the time or money for diabetes."
>
> SOURCE: Presented by Cohen Konrad, Pardue, and Hall, August 11, 2020.

centered on a 31-year-old woman with a variety of health concerns and barriers to care.[1] A full transcript of the video is presented in Box 4-2.

Cohen Konrad emphasized the importance of using case studies that learners can relate to in terms of culture and geography, and that resemble patients that the learners are likely to serve in their communities. However, she said, it is also important to be careful about perpetuating stereotypes and assumptions; using case studies can open up the discussion and allow instructors and learners to address these stereotypes. She said that the use of video can be extremely helpful because it gives learners a "visceral sense" of the client, and the ability to see the client in action. She noted, in response to a participant's question, that captions or transcripts can be used for videos in order to be accessible to those with hearing impairments. The discussion that followed is presented in Box 4-3.

The conscious instruction framework (see Figure 4-1), said Cohen Konrad, is multidimensional and intersectional, and it is designed "to hold us accountable as educators to teach and to create an environment for

---

[1] Hall, K. July 22, 2020. *Pat Chalmers case study*. UNE IPEC. https://www.youtube.com/watch?v=mVjii51ODzk (accessed November 28, 2020).

> **BOX 4-3**
> **Key Points Made by Individual Participants**
>
> A workshop participant queried others in the chat about diversity and inclusion by asking for strategies to engage students virtually who may require special auditory accommodations. Responses included
>
> - We had a student who was hearing impaired and got frustrated when video was used and ended up dropping out. The videos were captioned, but live remote communication was not optimal for this student. (Angie Portacio)
> - There is a captioning service/software for videos—a very important accommodation, and PowerPoint has a live captioning tool that can be broadcast over Zoom. Also regular check-ins with the student can help. (Valarie Fleming)
> - Provide closed captioning and transcripts of videos to assist students who have a hearing impairment. (Loretta Nunez)
> - Consider what happens in the classroom when students or educators with hearing impairments try to communicate with those wearing masks. (Melanie Bowzer)
> - For the remote learning and your students with hearing loss—if there is a group discussion, making sure all students in the discussion are enabling video while they talk can also help all students better follow the conversation. This is in addition to captions for videos—Microsoft Stream apparently automatically captions videos (i.e., prerecorded lectures). We have been dealing with this extensively in our audiology department where many of our students are hearing impaired and we serve patients with hearing loss. (Stephanie Fowler)
>
> SOURCE: Adapted from the presentation by Cohen Konrad, August 11, 2020.

learning." The framework includes three domains: content, context, and method. Content—the knowledge that is transferred—is "never neutral," said Cohen Konrad. There is a mythology, she said, that health education is based on facts and is on "neutral ground." To the contrary, nothing in education—content, context, or methods—is ever neutral. Content includes

- What definitions are used?
- Where does the evidence come from?
- What reflexive knowledge is being formally communicated?
- How does the instructor's own experience inform the teaching?
- What is the instructor's level of comfort with the material?

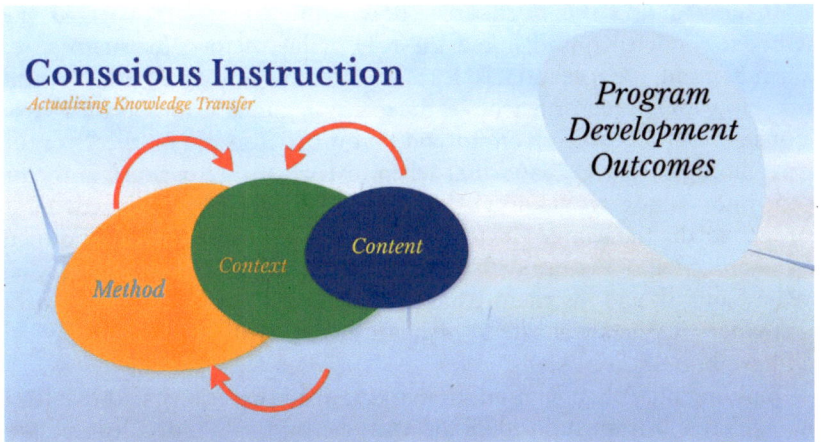

FIGURE 4-1 Conscious instruction framework.
SOURCE: Presented by Cohen Konrad, Pardue, and Hall, August 11, 2020.

Cohen Konrad went on to describe how effective teaching requires intellectual and emotional engagement risking exhaustion, disengagement, and burnout. It is the role of faculty and trainers to impart an understanding of self-awareness among their educators, she said, but according to Shealy et al. (2019), the trainers need to be self-aware and confident themselves before they can train others in the area of self-awareness. Pardue picked up on this notion saying that instructors have a responsibility to be self-reflective in their teaching, and to continuously assess and adapt their practice and the content based on inputs such as student, peer, or supervisor feedback, video recordings, and personal teaching notes. "Reflective teachers assume responsibility for continuously assessing the content … and actively considering the answer to the question, 'How am I doing in my teaching practice?'"

The next area Pardue covered involved the context in which education is delivered to, and received by, faculty and others. Context is influenced by multiple factors: by select critical and sociological theories, by what is included and excluded from the narrative, by implicit and explicit bias and assumptions, and by social determinants and individual circumstances. Considerations of context involve deliberate examination of power structures and decision-making practices, challenging the status quo, and giving voice to individuals and populations commonly not heard. Pardue encouraged participants to think back to the video case study and consider what unique circumstances and professional biases affected knowledge transfer in that example.

In considering the third area, how knowledge is transferred (i.e., methods), Cohen Konrad noted the role of instructors. Instructors, said Cohen Konrad, are role models; learners watch what they do and how they do it. How an instructor teaches is the method, and is as important as what he or she teaches. Cohen Konrad said that instructors are on the "frontline of psychological safety," and that when instructors are curious, authentic, open, and willing to acknowledge biases and missteps, they encourage learners to do the same. Health professional education involves difficult conversations about issues such as race, justice, and sexual orientation, said Cohen Konrad, and instructors have a responsibility to create an environment where learners feel safe to make mistakes, propose alternative views, and have honest discussions.

Building on Cohen Konrad's remarks, Pardue described affective learning. Affective learning considers the attitudes and values of a learner, with the goal of achieving a demonstrable change in a person's behavior. This type of teaching requires enormous creativity and use of multiple modalities, such as a video that draws the learner in visually and auditorily. A workshop participant asked how to assess whether methods such as video are useful. Cohen Konrad responded saying they use rapid cycle evaluation to gather input from learners about what methods are effective. At UNE, they also look at whether learners are achieving the goal competencies.

Power Dynamics

Before leaving the methods domain, Cohen Konrad acknowledged the need to discuss power. No matter the instructional method, she said, there are natural power dynamics. Instructors select the content, select the method, do the evaluating, and determine "whose story is told and whose story isn't told." Instructors decide whether to "radically listen and respond," or to instead cut off discussions that may be uncomfortable. Instructors need to engage with power dynamics, acknowledge power differentials, and engage students in these conversations, she said. Cohen Konrad suggested one way to flip this dynamic is to engage local communities in developing content, context, and method. For example, UNE worked with members of immigrant and refugee populations in Portland, Maine, to develop a course called "Empowering Cultural Education." The course was developed, taught, and evaluated by the community, along with an evaluation tool for measuring cultural competence and cultural humility. Cohen Konrad said that it was a "very critical learning experience" about teaching *with* populations, rather than *about* them.

Self-Awareness, Restoration, and Growth

The conscious instruction framework, said Cohen Konrad, also includes self-awareness, restoration, and growth as beneficial outcomes of using the model. Teaching, according to Bodenheimer and Shuster (2020), involves strenuous emotional labor and leaves instructors vulnerable to burnout and intellectual fatigue. A conscious instruction practice can help reduce burnout and increase the likelihood of instructor satisfaction, Cohen Konrad noted. *Self-awareness*, said Pardue, is a deliberate, conscious knowledge of ourselves, and involves focused attention and honesty in exploring the "why" of ideas, thoughts and actions. It provides faculty an opportunity to be objectively curious about themselves. Dedicating time and deliberate attention to self-awareness, said Pardue, leads to instructor restoration. *Restoration* is "the experience of feeling renewed and healed." Restoration liberates faculty, and it sparks creativity and new connections. A restorative state is reinvigorating, and it can serve as a buffer to the demanding, challenging work of teaching, she added. Finally, *growth* includes advancing our own knowledge, professional development, and instructional inspiration.

In many respects, Pardue noted, the conscious instruction framework parallels the quadruple aim of health care (Bodenheimer and Sinsky, 2014). These frameworks focus on improving quality (of education or care), improving the experience (of a learner or a patient), and assuring well-being (of instructors or health care providers). Pardue further noted that both frameworks can also reduce costs—if faculty are satisfied and reinvigorated with their work, they are less likely to leave.

Skilling Me Softly

In the closing minutes of the session, Pardue introduced participants to an exercise called "Skilling Me Softly" where she asked the participants to reflect back on the Pat case study (see Box 4-2). She then presented a list of desired qualities and skills for health care workers (see Box 4-4) and invited participants to think about how they would use the video case study to transfer knowledge of these assets. Pardue encouraged participants to continue thinking about how they would use the video, their comfort level in doing so, and what barriers might exist to achieving success (i.e., demonstrating acquisition of the desired skill or quality).

> **BOX 4-4**
> **Qualities and Skills for Current and Future Health Care Workers**
>
> - Critical thinking and curiosity
> - Cultural humility
> - Patient inclusion and responsivity
> - Problem solving
> - Collaboration and teamwork
> - Compassion and empathy
> - Communication skills
> - Adaptability
> - Collaborative leadership
>
> SOURCE: Presented by Pardue, August 11, 2020.

REFERENCES

Bodenheimer, G., and S. M. Shuster. 2020. Emotional labour, teaching and burnout: Investigating complex relationships. *Educational Research* 62(1):63–76.

Bodenheimer, T., and C. Sinsky. 2014. From triple to quadruple aim: Care of the patient requires care of the provider. *Annals of Family Medicine* 12(6):573–576.

Brown, B. 2018. *Dare to lead: Brave work. Tough conversations. Whole hearts.* New York: Penguin Random House.

Edmondson, A. C. 1999. Psychological safety and learning behavior in work teams. *Administrative Science Quarterly* 44(2):350–383.

Shealy, S. C., C. L. Worrall, J. L. Baker, A. D. Grant, P. H. Fabel, C. M. Walker, B. Ziegler, and W. D. Maxwell. 2019. Assessment of a faculty and preceptor development intervention to foster self-awareness and self-confidence. *American Journal of Pharmaceutical Education* 83(7):6920. https://doi.org/10.5688/ajpe6920.

Tobin, K. 2009. Tuning into others' voices: Radical listening, learning from difference, and escaping oppression. *Cultural Studies of Science Education* 4:505–511. https://doi.org/10.1007/s11422-009-9218-1.

5

Building Facilitating Structures for Informal Faculty Development (Step 4)

HIGHLIGHTS

- Some of the most profound insights can come from incidental and informal learning. (Sherman)
- Faculty should strive to create "learnable moments" when they are open to and aware of the potential for learning. (Sherman)

BUILDING FACILITATING STRUCTURES FOR INFORMAL (AND INCIDENTAL) FACULTY DEVELOPMENT

Lawrence Sherman, Meducate Global, LLC, and Association for Medical Education in Europe

"Informal and incidental learning does not mean unimportant learning," said Lawrence Sherman, principal of Meducate Global, LLC, and international development expert at the Association for Medical Education in Europe (AMEE). Learning can happen in any time or place, including a casual conversation, watching a movie, or reading a comic strip. Sherman said that while his presentation was focused specifically on faculty development, informal learning is a lifelong process for all people. For example, he said, finding and cultivating a prospective faculty member (i.e., pre-faculty development) could happen informally and incidentally, through a chance meeting or a casual conversation. While informal faculty development is the fourth step in the framework, he said that it is applicable to all of the other steps as well.

Sherman offered definitions for both *informal* and *incidental* learning, which are sometimes used interchangeably but are quite different. Informal learning, he said, is learning that happens outside a formal environment (e.g., classroom) but where there is still an expectation of learning. For example, informal learning could happen while reading articles, watching a webinar, listening to mentors, or talking with colleagues. Incidental learning, on the other hand, is learning that happens "when you don't expect it." These experiences can happen while watching television, talking with a passenger on a plane, looking at social media, or interacting with people outside one's own profession. For example, Sherman said, he has learned lessons from conversations with people ranging from oil executives to pilots about how to be a better teacher. He also noted that "there were no greater lessons learned about presenting to a challenging audience or a group of learners" than being a stand-up comic at 2:00 a.m. in a comedy club in New York—these lessons are engrained in him.

At the 2019 workshop Strengthening the Connection Between Health Professions Education and Practice, four broad themes were identified: technology, incentives and support, interprofessional continuing education, and communication. In all of these areas, said Sherman, one can see the value of informal and incidental education. He noted that informal education does not necessarily require financial resources, but it requires investing time in building a system that supports faculty in connecting with one another and allows for opportunities for informal learning. Sherman said there have been many times in his career when he learned lessons from a "conversation with somebody in the hallway," or talking to someone in a different profession who had a different perspective on practice or education. We encourage faculty to create "teachable moments" for students, he said, but faculty also need to strive to find "learnable moments" for themselves. Sherman asked participants in a poll whether informal and incidental learning are important to faculty development. Some participants chose "Yes, of course!" while others chose "Yes, but it only happens when it happens."

Is it possible, asked Sherman, to be *intentionally* incidental and informal? In the context of learning, a learner can be guided, with the objectives controlled by the teacher, or a learner can be the discoverer and in control of the learning objectives (see Figure 5-1). The beauty of informal and incidental learning, said Sherman, is that it is unstructured, unplanned, unexpected, and the learner identifies their own opportunities for new skills and knowledge. However, it is possible to be intentional in encouraging faculty to discover things on their own. Intentionally encouraging and supporting informal learning can help identify, support, and retain faculty, he said. For example, faculty can be encouraged to intentionally identify skills or knowledge that they need, and to find "learnable moments" to develop these.

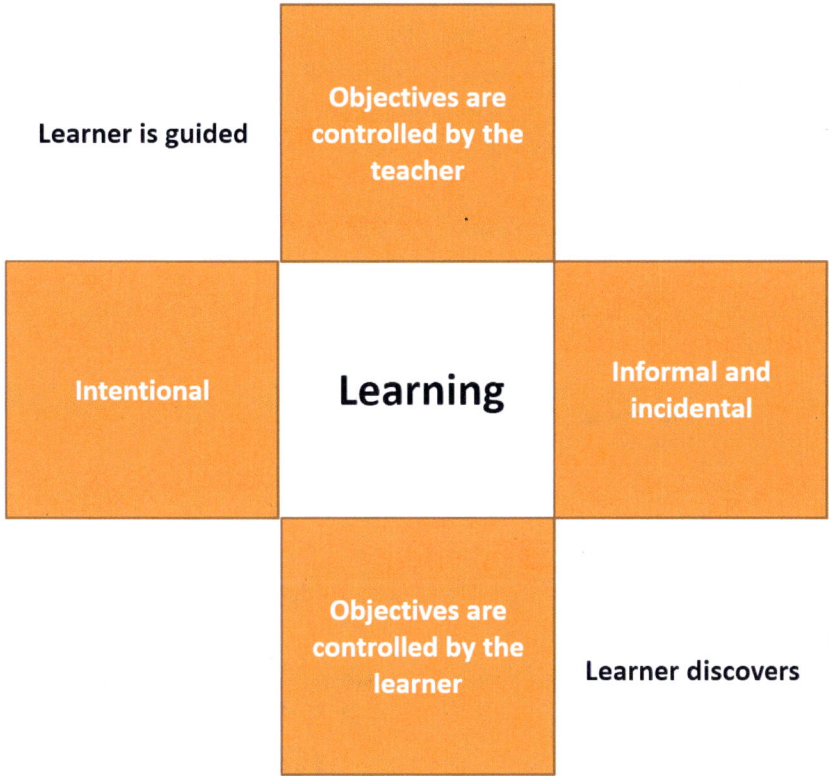

FIGURE 5-1 Matrix of learning.
SOURCE: Presented by Sherman, August 11, 2020.

Workshop participants offered ideas in the chat box about how informal and incidental learning could be supported and facilitated (see Box 5-1). Chappell noted that recognizing and reflecting on incidental learning is a skill, and wondered if this skill could be strengthened in faculty. Poll-Hunter said that for informal and incidental learning to be effective, faculty "need to be comfortable with being uncomfortable and being inconvenienced." Kylie Dotson-Blake concurred and added that successful education requires seeing learners as people "who bring their whole selves, their full complexities of context and intersections of identity and experiences into the learning community." Participants mentioned faculty book clubs, the use of "near-peer" mentors for guidance and training, brown bag lunches, volunteering, and community engagement. Artino brought up "water cooler learning," and Sherman noted that this type of informal learning could

> **BOX 5-1**
> **Key Points Made by Individual Participants**
>
> Chappell asked participants to reflect on how they might create opportunities for informal and incidental learning within their own settings. Responses included
>
> - In pre-COVID, conversations traveling on the way to places; having leaners over to house, breaking bread. COVID makes the things we do on the way to other things go away. How do we recreate these opportunities under COVID? (Warren Newton)
> - I learn so much from my peer faculty through informal conversations. (Lori Greene)
> - This chat box is a great example of our current COVID-19 strategies to learn from each other. (Norma Poll-Hunter)
> - I sometimes notice certain faculty are quicker to recognize that incidental learning has occurred—pause and reflect on it. Is that a skill (this insight) we can strengthen to boost the impact of this type of learning? (Reamer Bushardt)
> - Incidental learning can occur through reading student feedback, in assignments, discussions. (Kathy Chappell)
> - We had success from signposting informal/incidental learning—helping learners identify, record, and enhance their own learning. (Warren Newton)
> - An example of good informal learning might occur when faculty attend professional meetings and network with other professionals working in the field. (Sandra)
> - The breaks at a meeting might be just as important as the meeting itself. (Patricia Cuff)
> - Opportunities depend greatly on the teaching and learning styles of different cultures. (Ying-Chiao Tsao)
> - It seems to me that educators need to be comfortable with being uncomfortable and being inconvenienced—they never know what a learner will share or an unexpected question that may be asked. (Norma Poll-Hunter)
>
> SOURCE: Adapted from the presentation by Sherman, August 11, 2020.

even take place virtually, with a weekly informal video chat between colleagues. Poll-Hunter mentioned that the chat box itself was an example of an environment for informal learning.

To close, Sherman showed participants a framework for informal and incidental learning that was developed by Marsick and Watkins and later modified by Cseh et al. (1998) (see Figure 5-2). The model describes the process of workplace learning based on a trigger occurring in a specific context, followed by problem solving and ongoing reflection (Marsick et al.,

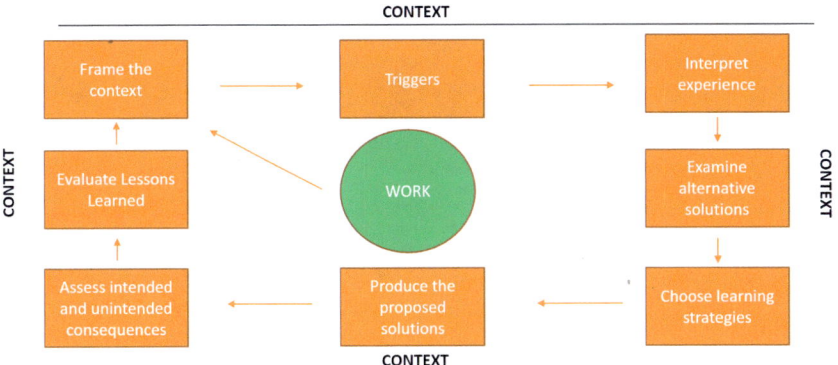

FIGURE 5-2 Framework for informal and incidental learning.
SOURCES: Presented by Sherman, August 11, 2020; Cseh et al., 2000; Marsick and Watkins, 1990.

2006). Sherman encouraged workshop participants to consider how they might incorporate such a framework into their own faculty development efforts before handing the microphone over to Poll-Hunter.

Poll-Hunter thanked Sherman for calling attention to those learnable moments in everyday life to maximize our own informal education. With that, Poll-Hunter moved to the final session.

REFERENCES

Cseh, M., K. Watkins, and V. Marsick. 2000. Informal and incidental learning in the workplace. In *Conceptions of self-directed learning, theoretical and conceptual considerations.* Edited by G. A. Straka. New York: Waxman. Pp. 59–74.
Marsick, V. J., and K. E. Watkins. 1990. *Informal and incidental learning in the workplace.* London, UK: Routledge.
Marsick, V., K. E. Watkins, M. Callahan, and M. Volpe. 2006. *Reviewing theory and research on informal and incidental learning.* https://files.eric.ed.gov/fulltext/ED492754.pdf (accessed December 27, 2020).

6

Closing Reflections

HIGHLIGHTS

- Informal and incidental mentorship, especially of diverse learners, can help set learners on a path toward faculty careers. (Williams)
- Formal faculty development should include opportunities for self-reflection and consideration of learning objectives and priorities. (Williams)
- Faculty can leverage the learning potential of any situation by actively seeking out different people and perspectives. (Williams)
- The process of engaging with diverse people, settings, and experiences can expand and shift faculty's knowledge, skills, and aptitudes; this increases competence. (Williams)
- Double-loop learning can be a way to reconsider the traditional approach to faculty development. (Williams)

The last session of the workshop served to bring together threads from the other sessions and explicitly highlight diversity, equity, and inclusion in the steps of faculty development (see Figure 6-1). Norma Poll-Hunter, Association of American Medical Colleges (AAMC), introduced the session saying, "We've worked through each of the steps, and now what we want to do is underscore how diversity, equity, and inclusion are important threads in our work." Poll-Hunter further described the concepts of diversity and inclusion mentioned throughout all the presentations. The speakers encouraged everyone to explore their own responsibilities for preparing individuals to be culturally responsive and environmentally sensitive to

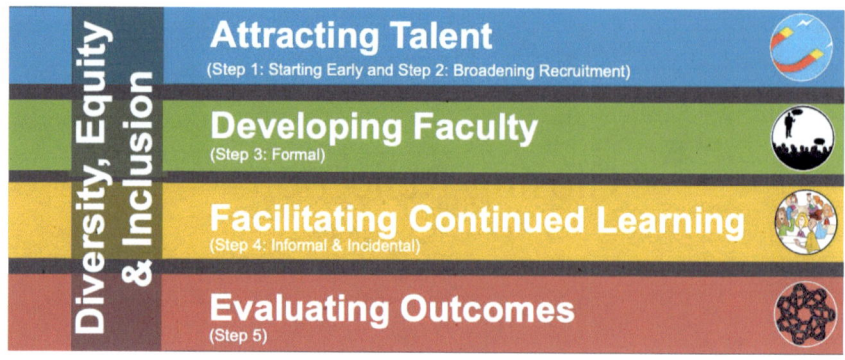

FIGURE 6-1 Framework for faculty development.
SOURCE: Presented by Williams, August 11, 2020.

the unique abilities of each learner. Participants were encouraged to think very broadly about diversity, inclusion, and equity as they listened to Valerie Williams reflect on the messages she heard through the lens of her experiences.

REFLECTIONS ON SPEAKERS' REMARKS

Valerie N. Williams, University of Oklahoma Health Sciences Center

Valerie Williams, vice provost for academic affairs and faculty development at the University of Oklahoma Health Sciences Center, summarized the "pearls" of wisdom from each session, offered her own perspective, and asked participants to share their insights in the chat box.

Attracting Talent

Attracting talented future health professions educators means starting early and broadening recruitment, said Williams. Sánchez had noted that the faculty of health professions education is not as diverse as it should be, and she said that there was a need for more intentional engagement with prospective faculty. Williams reflected on her own career, and said that both intentional and incidental mentors set her on the path into academic medicine. She encouraged participants to think more broadly about the idea of mentorship, and emphasized that "little *m*" mentoring can be as influential as "big *M*" mentoring. For example, faculty can reach out to pre-faculty learners through actions as small as an encouraging conversation or an invitation to an event. These types of informal interactions may be particularly

CLOSING REFLECTIONS 43

important, said Williams, to learners who are underrepresented in the environment. She encouraged participants to consider ways to invest in various forms of mentoring, and to select mentees who may not traditionally have health professions opportunities or mentors.

In reflecting on the other presentations, Williams described what she heard as four components in the ways connections are made and pathways are laid into health professions education (see Figure 6-2). Everything, she said, from engaging with student interest groups to understanding and talking about the benefits of being a health educator with learners, can potentially seed an opportunity. Opportunities also come from working with staff who are based in the community or in settings outside of the formal education setting, where there are other kinds of connections. Helping learners, whoever they are, pre-faculty or early-career educator-clinicians, to build an identity as an educator and then ultimately as a practitioner can open the way for mentoring someone who is underrepresented in the profession and on the faculty.

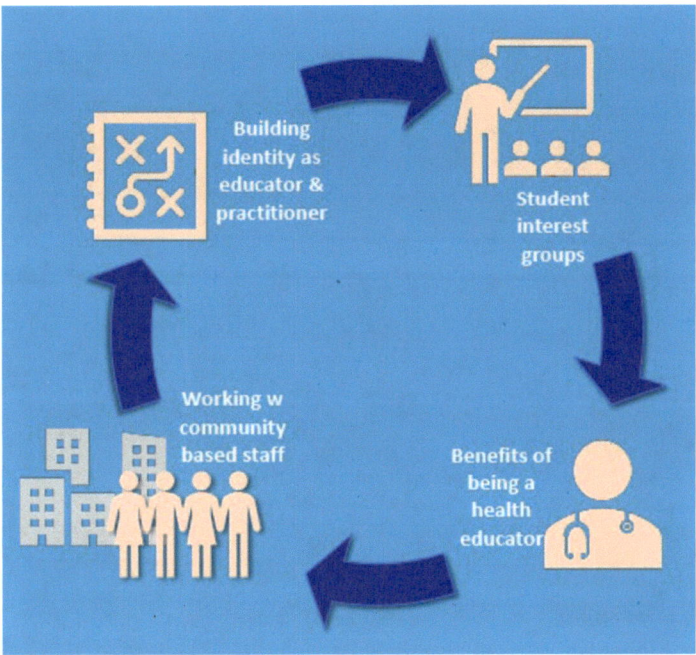

FIGURE 6-2 Mentoring relationships.
SOURCE: Presented by Williams, August 11, 2020.

Developing Faculty

Developing future health professions educators means offering current and new faculty formal opportunities for learning how to become more effective as an educator. Williams appreciated that Cohen Konrad, Hall, and Pardue used the term *aspirations* when presenting on the conscious instruction framework, because what learners aspire to may be very different, depending on their individual background, community, and culture. In formal faculty development, she said, learners are often told what they are expected to learn, rather than engaging in self-reflection about their own expectations and objectives. Faculty development should instead be an invitation to direct attention to different areas and to critically reflect on priorities and goals.

Williams developed Figure 6-3 in order to demonstrate the areas to which attention can be directed, and where shifts can be made to think and learn differently. For example, focusing on "place" by taking learning out of the typical classroom environment and into the community can give new insight into what patients are experiencing. An important area for reflection, said Williams, is to consider how educational institutions or workplaces can help faculty pay attention to issues such as engagement,

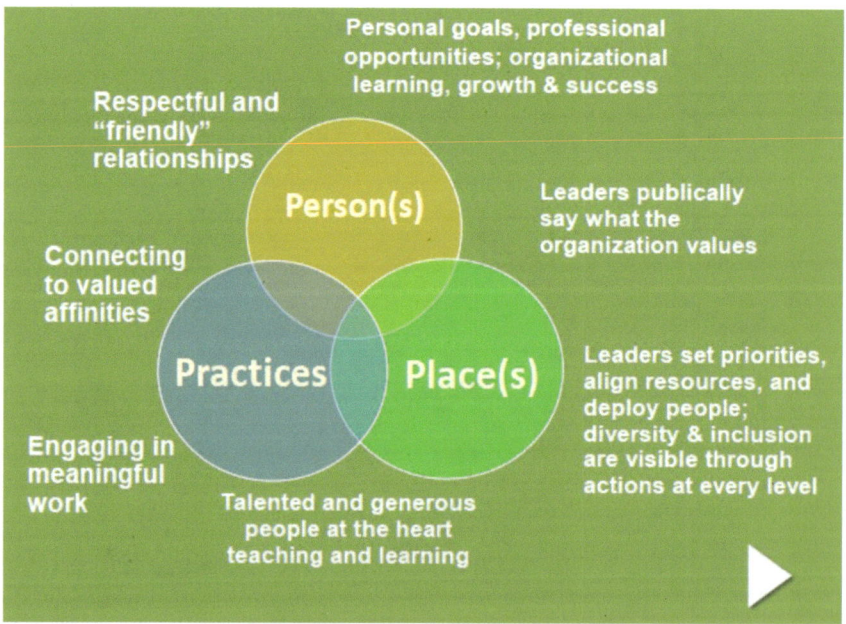

FIGURE 6-3 Directed attention.
SOURCE: Presented by Williams, August 11, 2020.

teamwork, impact, diversity, and transparency and accountability to the community.

Facilitating Continued Learning

Facilitating continued learning includes attending to informal and incidental learning opportunities for future health professions educators to enhance their knowledge, skills, and aptitudes. Williams said that Sherman's point about looking for "learnable moments" really resonated with her, and that "we can learn from not only the surroundings, but how we attend to the surroundings." That is, faculty can leverage the learning potential of any situation by actively seeking out different people and perspectives. Engaging with diverse people, settings, and experiences can expand and shift faculty's knowledge, skills, and aptitudes, she said, giving four examples:

1. Interprofessional teaching and learning allows us to hear from a broader array of individuals and professions;
2. Working with diverse or underrepresented community partners allows us to tap into new perspectives and collaborate on shared goals;
3. Community-based participatory research can be an avenue for building affinity-based relationships outside of the formal educational environment; and
4. Co-teaching with former patients can bring new insight about what a patient would want learners to understand about an acute or chronic illness.

Williams discussed her experience of working with community partners as a way to illuminate the potential for incidental learning opportunities. Williams is the director of a university center for excellence in developmental disabilities. One of the center's goals is to build a bridge between the university and people with developmental disabilities, families, providers, and other supports in the community. As part of this work, there is a community advisory group. When this group came together, Williams said, it was "not a symphony of voices but somewhat of a cacophony." There were widely different expectations of what the group would do, and different expectations of the partners within the group. Out of this cacophony came a list of 148 things that people wanted out of the partnership. The group engaged in long discussions about their values, expectations, and reasons for partnering, and ended up whittling the list down to seven values to guide their work:

1. Recognize the need to partner.
2. Value and respect each other.
3. Accept each other.
4. Set clear expectations.
5. Provide feedback.
6. Expect impact, product, or outcome.
7. Trust each other.

As important as the list of seven values is, said Williams, just as significant was the process work of engagement that went into it. The process, she said, is "what enables us to build the knowledge that lets us leverage the skills and the aptitudes within any group ... trying to achieve a common endpoint."

Evaluating Outcomes

Evaluating outcomes based on thoughtful program designs means beginning with a clear idea of the desired outcome, summarized Williams. The knowledge-to-action framework that Thomas and Artino presented was helpful because "nothing will happen if we are not enabled to act on good ideas." Using such a framework gives an opportunity to "test the waters" and to build a foundation for a "bigger and healthier house for the future." Being thoughtful about building this foundation is enormously important, because "we need many people to be able to walk that path and build and live in that house." The future health professions faculty hold the promise for all of us of a healthier society and healthier outcomes for people who are struggling with illness. Building this future is a "remarkable task" but one that is doable, Williams said.

Several presenters, said Williams, had touched on the importance of reflection at all stages of faculty development. Faculty development sometimes feels like a "vicious cycle" in which people are trying to change something but without any clear direction or forethought. She compared it to a group of people "rowing in every possible direction" and creating chaos and confusion by not asking where are *we* trying to go? In contrast, a "virtuous cycle" leads in the direction of positive change and alignment of a shared set of values. It requires reflective and active conversation, reflection about the actions taken and whether they will lead to the desired outcome, and listening to diverse voices. The idea of a "virtuous cycle" is similar to the concept of "double-loop learning," first described by Chris Argyris in 1991 (see Figure 6-4). Double-loop learning, said Williams, asks people to take a step back and consider the assumptions that underlie a plan of action, rather than simply adjusting the plan itself. There are certain things that are known about faculty development, including various approaches, how

CLOSING REFLECTIONS

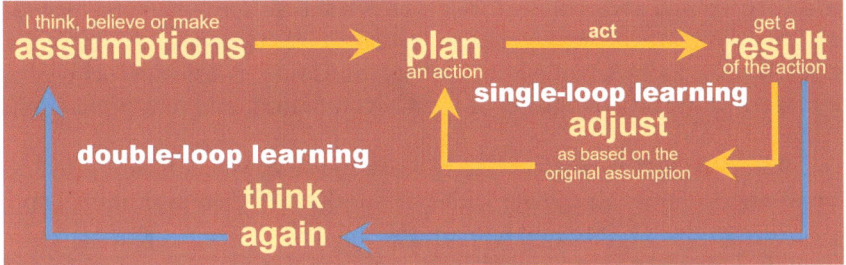

FIGURE 6-4 Double-loop learning.
SOURCES: Presented by Williams, August 11, 2020; adapted from Argyris, 1991.

it works, and for whom it works. "As we try to think about how to engage diverse audiences" in faculty development, said Williams, we should take the opportunity to step back and consider changing the way things have traditionally been done in order to do it better.

Finding the North Star in a Time of COVID

Chappell revisited her opening remarks by asking Williams what is her "north star." In other words, "What would be an actionable step that each of us could take within our own environment to move forward with thinking about what that north star might look like?" Williams responded by describing what she asks of her leaders and of herself—to have at least one conversation a week with someone you do not know, to ask them for perspective. She also acknowledged how personal networks have changed during the pandemic but that everyone at the university remains united behind fighting a common enemy, the coronavirus. However, she added, the thing about being in it together is we are still faced with a wide power and financial differential between, for example, the academic scholars and the cleaning staff. So to be in it together educators have to think about that full continuum of people and ask whether everybody is afforded similar access to information they can use, because that is part of those building blocks.

Closing Thoughts

In her concluding remarks, Williams said that health professions educators are like a symphony; each person must play his or her individual instruments, but together they can create beautiful music. Every individual is responsible for developing his or her own skills and bringing his or her personal, intellectual, and experiential capital to the table. Collectively, they can harmonize the work, collaborate, and advance the principles of diversity, equity, and inclusion as a powerful asset for achieving a shared aim. She invited workshop participants to consider what they would do differently after today's workshop, both as individual "musicians" as well as members of the broader group of faculty, community, and interprofessional teams.

Williams further emphasized the importance of giving faculty unstructured opportunities to engage with one another—"when everything is not structured down to the last hair on the nit, they share some remarkable insights." She noted that some faculty may find this easier than others, and suggested that various methods, such as virtual meetings or chat boxes, could be used to facilitate the broadest conversation. Williams said these kinds of open conversations can give faculty a chance to step back from their usual role as experts and allow them to see other perspectives and gain other insights. Williams added that faculty and learners all can benefit from talking to people "they don't usually talk to." Leaders in particular should seek out conversations with those outside of usual networks, communities, and circles, and invite people to speak "who have not spoken before."

PULLING IT ALL TOGETHER: REFLECTIONS ON THE STEPS

Reamer Bushardt, The George Washington University, and Kathy Chappell, American Nurses Credentialing Center

Bushardt and Chappell then closed the workshop with a look to the future. They expressed sentiments of hope that as the forum and today's participants have identified the kinds of skills and capabilities that our future workforce needs, the health professional educational and practice communities can work together across disciplines, learn from each other, and build momentum toward greater diversity, inclusiveness, and equity. Bushardt emphasized a point made by Williams that coming together around shared values for this work will ensure we are not all rowing in different directions but all heading together toward that "north star."

REFERENCE

Argyris, C. 1991. Teaching smart people how to learn. *Harvard Business Review*, May–June. https://hbr.org/1991/05/teaching-smart-people-how-to-learn (accessed December 16, 2020).

Appendix A

Members of the Global Forum on Innovation in Health Professional Education[1,2]

Caswell A. Evans, D.D.S., M.P.H. (*Co-Chair*)
NAM Member
Associate Dean for Prevention and Public Health Services
University of Illinois at Chicago College of Dentistry

Deborah Powell, M.D. (*Co-Chair*)
NAM Member
Professor, Department of Laboratory Medicine and Pathology
University of Minnesota

Frank J. Ascione, Pharm.D., M.P.H., Ph.D.
Director, University of Michigan Center for Interprofessional Education
Professor of Clinical and Social and Administrative Sciences
University of Michigan College of Pharmacy
Michigan Center for Interprofessional Education

David Benton, R.G.N., Ph.D., FFNF, FRCN, FAAN
Chief Executive Officer
National Council of State Boards of Nursing

---

[1] The National Academies of Sciences, Engineering, and Medicine's forums and roundtables do not issue, review, or approve individual documents. The responsibility for the published Proceedings of a Workshop rests with the workshop rapporteurs and the institution.

[2] Forum sponsors and in-kind donators identified in italic.

Mary Jo Bondy, D.H.Ed., M.H.S., PA-C
Chief Executive Officer
Physician Assistant Education Association

Reamer L. Bushardt, Pharm.D., PA-C, DFAAPA
Senior Associate Dean for Health Sciences
The George Washington University

Robert Cain, D.O.
Chief Executive Officer
American Association of Colleges of Osteopathic Medicine

Kathy Chappell, Ph.D., R.N., FNAP, FAAN
Senior Vice President
Certification/Measurement, Accreditation, and Institute for Credentialing Research
American Nurses Credentialing Center

Steven Chesbro, P.T., D.P.T., Ed.D.
Vice President for Education
American Physical Therapy Association

Amy Aparicio Clark, M.Ed.
Senior Program Officer, Cultivating Healthy Communities
Aetna Foundation

Darla Spence Coffey, M.S.W., Ph.D.
President
Council on Social Work Education

Darrin D'Agostino, D.O., M.P.H., M.B.A.
Executive Dean and Vice President of Health Affairs
Kansas City University of Medicine and Biosciences
American Association of Colleges of Osteopathic Medicine

Jan de Maeseneer, M.D., Ph.D., FRCGP (Hon)
Chairman for European Forum for Primary Care Secretary-General
The Network: Towards Unity for Health
Vice-Dean for Strategic Planning at the Faculty of Medicine and Health Science
Ghent University (Belgium)

APPENDIX A

Marietjie de Villiers, Ph.D., M.B.Ch.B., M.Fam.Med., FCFP
Professor in Family Medicine
Deputy Dean, Education
Stellenbosch University

Kylie P. Dotson-Blake, Ph.D., NCC, LPC
President and Chief Executive Officer
NBCC, Inc., and Affiliates

Kim Dunleavy, Ph.D., MOMT, P.T., OCS
Associate Clinical Professor
Director, Professional Education and Community Engagement
Department of Physical Therapy
University of Florida
American Council of Academic Physical Therapy

Kathrin (Katie) Eliot, Ph.D., R.D.
Director
Health Professions Educator
University of Oklahoma Health Sciences Center
Academy of Nutrition and Dietetics

Sara E. Fletcher, Ph.D.
Vice President and Chief Learning Officer
Interim Chief Executive Officer
Physician Assistant Education Association

Jody Frost, P.T., D.P.T., Ph.D., FAPTA, FNAP
President-Elect
National Academies of Practice

Elizabeth (Liza) Goldblatt, Ph.D., M.P.A./H.A.
Director of Planning and Assessment
American College of Traditional Chinese Medicine
Board Chair
Academic Collaborative for Integrative Health

Catherine L. Grus, Ph.D.
Deputy Executive Director for Education
American Psychological Association

Anita Gupta, D.O., Pharm.D., M.P.P.
Senior Vice President, Medical Strategy & Government Affairs
Heron Therapeutics, Inc.

Kendra Harrington, P.T., D.P.T., M.S.
Board-Certified Clinical Specialist in Women's Health Physical Therapy
Director, Residency/Fellowship Accreditation
American Board of Physical Therapy Residency and Fellowship Education
American Physical Therapy Association

Neil Harvison, Ph.D., OTR/L, FAOTA
Chief Academic and Scientific Affairs Officer
American Occupational Therapy Association

Eric Holmboe, M.D.
Senior Vice President
Milestones Development and Evaluation
Accreditation Council for Graduate Medical Education

Lisa Howley, M.Ed., Ph.D.
Senior Director of Strategic Initiatives and Partnerships
Association of American Medical Colleges

Holly Humphrey, M.D.
President
Josiah Macy Jr. Foundation

Emilia Iwu, M.S.N., R.N., APNC, FWACN
Ph.D. Scholar
Rutgers University

Pamela Jeffries, Ph.D., R.N., FAAN, ANEF
Dean of Nursing
The George Washington University

Phyllis M. King, Ph.D., OT, FAOTA, FASAHP
Associate Vice Chancellor for Academic Affairs, University of Wisconsin–Milwaukee
Chair
Association of Schools of the Allied Health Professions

APPENDIX A

Sandeep "Sunny" Kishore, M.D., Ph.D., M.Sc.
President
Young Professionals Chronic Disease Network
Associate Director, Arnhold Institute for Global Health
Icahn School of Medicine at Mount Sinai

Kathleen Klink, M.D., FAAFP
Chief of Health Professions Education
Office of Academic Affiliations, Veterans Health Administration

Kathryn (Kathy) Kolasa, Ph.D., RDN, LDN
Professor Emeritus and Master Educator Department of Family Medicine-
    Nutrition and Patient Education
East Carolina University Brody School of Medicine
Academy of Nutrition and Dietetics

Kimberly Lomis, M.D.
Vice President for Undergraduate Medical Education Innovations
American Medical Association

Chao Ma, M.D.
Dean of Medical Education
Peking Union Medical College
Chinese Academy of Medical Sciences

Andrew Maccabe, D.V.M.
Executive Director
Association of American Veterinary Medical Colleges

Beverly Malone, Ph.D., R.N., FAAN
NAM Member
Chief Executive Officer
National League for Nursing

Mary E. (Beth) Mancini, R.N., Ph.D., N.E.-B.C., FAHA, ANEF, FAAN
Associate Dean and Chair, Undergraduate Nursing Programs
Baylor Professor for Healthcare Research
The University of Texas at Arlington
College of Nursing
Past President
Society for Simulation in Healthcare

Dawn M. Mancuso, MAM, CAE, FASAE
Executive Director
Association of Schools and Colleges of Optometry

Angelo McClain, Ph.D., LICSW
Chief Executive Officer
National Association of Social Workers

Lemmietta G. McNeilly, Ph.D., CCC-SLP, CAE
Chief Staff Officer, Speech-Language Pathology
ASHA Fellow
American Speech-Language-Hearing Association

Mark Merrick, Ph.D., ATC, FNATA
Past President
Commission on Accreditation of Athletic Training Education
Athletic Training Strategic Alliance

Suzanne Miyamoto, Ph.D., R.N., FAAN
Chief Executive Officer
American Academy of Nursing

Warren Newton, M.D., M.P.H.
President and Chief Executive Officer Elect
American Board of Family Medicine

Loretta Nunez, M.A., Au.D., CCC-A/SLP, FNAP
ASHA Fellow
Director of Academic Affairs & Research Education
American Speech-Language-Hearing Association

David O'Bryon, J.D., CAE
President
Association of Chiropractic Colleges
Immediate-Past Chair
Academic Collaborative for Integrative Health

Bjorg Palsdottir, M.P.A.
Executive Director and Co-Founder
Training for Health Equity Network

APPENDIX A

Miguel Paniagua, M.D.
Medical Advisor, Test Materials Development
National Board of Medical Examiners

Rajata Rajatanavin, M.D., FAC
Minister of Public Health
Government of Thailand

Thomas Rebbecchi, M.D.
Medical Advisor, Marketing and Product Management
National Board of Medical Examiners

Jo Ann Regan, Ph.D., M.S.W.
Vice President of Education
Council on Social Work Education

Lucy A. Savitz, Ph.D., M.B.A.
Vice President, Research
Director, Center for Health Research, Oregon | Hawaii
Kaiser Permanente

Stephen Schoenbaum, M.D., M.P.H.
Special Advisor to the President
Josiah Macy Jr. Foundation

Joanne G. Schwartzberg, M.D.
Scholar-in-Residence
Accreditation Council for Graduate Medical Education

Wendi Schweiger, Ph.D., NCC, LPC
Director, NBCC International Capacity Building
Foundation and Professional Services
National Board for Certified Counselors, Inc., & Affiliates

Nelson Sewankambo, M.B.Ch.B., M.Sc., M.Med., FRCP Doctor of Laws (HC)
NAM Member
Principal and Professor
Makerere University College of Health Sciences

Javaid I. Sheikh, M.D., M.B.A.
Dean
Weill Cornell Medicine–Qatar

Carl J. Sheperis, Ph.D.
Dean, College of Education and Human Development
Texas A&M University–San Antonio

Susan E. Skochelak, M.D., M.P.H.
NAM Member
Vice President, Medical Education
American Medical Association

Jeffrey Stewart, D.D.S., M.S.
Senior Vice President for Interprofessional and Global Collaboration
American Dental Education Association

Zohray Talib, M.D.
Senior Associate Dean for Academic Engagement and Chair of Medical Education
California University of Science and Medicine

Maria Tassone, M.Sc.
Senior Director, Health Professions and Interprofessional Care, University Health Network
Director, Centre for Interprofessional Education, University of Toronto
University of Toronto and University Health Network/Michener Institute of Education

Melissa Trego, D.O., Ph.D.
Dean
Salus University, Pennsylvania College of Optometry
Association of Schools and Colleges of Optometry

Carole Tucker, Ph.D., M.S.
Associate Professor in the College of Public Health and the College of Engineering
Temple University
American Council of Academic Physical Therapy

Richard Weisbarth, O.D., FAAO, FNAP
Vice President, Professional Affairs for CIBA Vision Corporation
Alcon
President-Elect
National Academies of Practice

Karen P. West, D.M.D., M.P.H.
President and Chief Executive Officer
American Dental Education Association

Alison J. Whelan, M.D.
Chief Medical Education Officer
Association of American Medical Colleges

Adrienne White-Faines, M.P.A.
Chief Executive Officer
American Osteopathic Association

Launette Woolforde, Ed.D., DNP, R.N.-BC
Nursing Education and Professional Development, Northwell Health
National League for Nursing

Xuejun Zeng, M.D., Ph.D., FACP
Chief and Associate Chair
Division of General Internal Medicine, Peking Union Medical College Department of Medicine
Chinese Academy of Medical Sciences

Board on Global Health and Global Forum on Innovation in Health Professional Education Staff

Julie Pavlin, M.D., Ph.D., M.P.H.
Senior Director
Board on Global Health

Patricia Cuff, M.P.H., M.S.
Forum Director and Senior Program Officer
Board on Global Health

Hannah Goodtree
Research Assistant
Board on Global Health

Appendix B

Workshop Agenda

August 11, 2020
Online

HEALTH PROFESSIONS FACULTY FOR THE FUTURE

OPENING SESSION

Session Objective: To review five steps to an effective faculty as gleaned from the previous forum workshop Strengthening the Connection Between Health Professions Education and Practice

11:00 a.m.   **Welcome and orientation to the workshop**
Workshop co-chairs: Reamer Bushardt, The George Washington University (GWU), and Kathy Chappell, American Nurses Credentialing Center (ANCC)

    Summary of needs assessment
Lawrence Sherman, Meducate Global, LLC, and Association for Medical Education in Europe (AMEE)

FIVE STEPS TO BUILD THE FACULTY OF THE FUTURE

11:25 a.m.	Each speaker will state why the step is important and how can it be applied. Moderators: Reamer Bushardt, GWU, and Kathy Chappell, ANCC
11:30 a.m.	**STEP 5: Evaluate effects of a faculty development program using a framework or model** Starting with the end in mind: Designing and evaluating faculty development Anthony Artino, GWU, and Aliki Thomas, McGill University
12:00–12:15 p.m.	[15 min intermission—do not exit the webinar]
12:15 p.m.	**STEP 1: Start early building a pipeline into education** **STEP 2: Broaden recruitment into health professions education** Diversity and inclusion into health professions education Moderator: Norma Poll-Hunter, Association of American Medical Colleges (AAMC) John-Paul Sánchez, University of New Mexico
12:50 p.m.	**STEP 3: Train new recruits and current faculty to be effective educators** Formal faculty development for building critical educator skill sets Shelley Cohen Konrad, University of New England (UNE); Karen Pardue, UNE; and Kris Hall, UNE
1:20 p.m.	**STEP 4: Build facilitating structures for informal faculty development** Informal faculty development Lawrence Sherman, Meducate Global, LLC, and AMEE

PULLING IT ALL TOGETHER

1:50 p.m.	**Closing reflections**
	Diversity and inclusion
	    Moderator: Norma Poll-Hunter, AAMC
	    Valerie N. Williams, University of Oklahoma Health Sciences Center

2:20 p.m.	**Pulling it all together: Reflections on the steps** Workshop co-chairs: Reamer Bushardt, GWU, and Kathy Chappell, ANCC
2:30 p.m.	**ADJOURN**

Appendix C

Speaker Biographical Sketches

Reamer L. Bushardt, Pharm.D., PA-C, DFAAPA (*Workshop Co-Chair*), is a tenured educator, researcher, clinician, and administrator with experience in rural, community-based practice and with faculty service within three academic medical centers. He is a professor and a senior associate dean in the School of Medicine and Health Sciences at The George Washington University (GWU) in Washington, DC. In this role, he oversees departments and centers comprising more than 40 programs in the health professions and translational sciences. He is licensed as a physician assistant and a pharmacist and has specialized training and experience in caring for patients with emphasis on management of chronic illness and interventions to address inappropriate polypharmacy and drug injury. He regularly teaches and mentors trainees in the areas of pharmacology and clinical research. He is the principal investigator for the George Washington Health Careers Opportunity Program, a health care workforce development program funded by the U.S. Health Resources and Services Administration. He is the director of the Translational Workforce Development in the Clinical Translational Science Institute—Children's Network (CTSI-CN), funded by the National Institutes of Health's National Center for Advancing Translational Science. The CTSI-CN is a partnership between the Children's National Health System and GWU. Dr. Bushardt is a director-at-large on the board of the Physician Assistant Education Association. He is the editor-in-chief emeritus for the *Journal of the American Academy of Physician Assistants*. He previously served as a department chair at the Wake Forest School of Medicine and as the associate vice president for workforce innovation at the Wake Forest Baptist Medical Center in Winston-Salem, North Carolina. He was also an associate professor and a division chief for physician assistant studies at the Medical University of South Carolina in Charleston.

Kathy Chappell, Ph.D., R.N., FNAP, FAAN (*Workshop Co-Chair*), is the senior vice president of certification, measurement, accreditation, and research at the American Nurses Credentialing Center. She is responsible for the certification of individual registered nurses and advanced practice registered nurses, as well as the development of certification examinations. She is responsible for the accreditation of organizations that provide continuing nursing education and interprofessional continuing education and for the accreditation of residency and fellowship programs for nurses. She also directs the Institute for Credentialing Research, analyzing outcomes related to credentialing. She holds a baccalaureate in nursing with distinction from the University of Virginia, a master of science in advanced clinical nursing, and a doctorate in nursing from George Mason University. She is a fellow in the American Academy of Nursing and a distinguished scholar and a fellow in the National Academies of Practice.

Anthony R. Artino, Jr., Ph.D., is a tenured professor of health, human function, and rehabilitation sciences at The George Washington University (GWU) School of Medicine and Health Sciences. He received his Ph.D. in educational psychology from the University of Connecticut and accrued more than 23 years of leadership experience as a captain in the U.S. Navy prior to his arrival at GWU. In his current role, he teaches graduate courses, conducts research, mentors students and junior faculty, and provides administrative leadership in evaluation and educational research. As a researcher, he has been the principal or the associate investigator on more than $8 million in funded research. His most highly cited works are a blend of research and education articles on topics ranging from analyzing and interpreting survey data, understanding academic motivation and self-regulated learning among medical students and practicing physicians, measuring long-term physician outcomes, and developing questionnaires for educational research. Dr. Artino is a deputy editor for the *Journal of Graduate Medical Education* and an assistant editor for *Academic Medicine*. He is also a fellow of the Association for Medical Education in Europe. He has published 200 scientific articles and book chapters and conducted 150 invited talks, research presentations, and conference workshops on learning and assessment for international audiences around the globe.

Shelley Cohen Konrad, Ph.D., LCSW, FNAP, is the director of and a professor in the School of Social Work and the director of the Center for Excellence in Collaborative Education (CECE). A clinical social worker by training, Dr. Cohen Konrad specializes in practice with children and families. The second edition of her book, *Practice with Children and Families: A Relational Perspective*, was published in December 2019. In 1988 Dr. Cohen Konrad established Touchstone Psychotherapy Associates, a mental health collaborative designed to meet the complex needs of children, families, and carers. She co-founded the Kids First Center in 1997, a Portland-based, nonprofit program serving children, parenting partners, and families experiencing divorce, family disruption, and parental separation. Dr. Cohen Konrad is committed to improving the quality of health and health-related care for all people. In 2010 she was named founding director of the University of New England's Interprofessional Education Collaborative (IPEC) and in 2019 IPEC was named as a Center for Excellence in Collaborative Education. CECE designs and implements educational programming that brings together students and faculty to learn about, from, and with each other. The purpose of shared learning is to prepare graduates to be both excellent in their chosen fields as well as proficient members of practice teams. The overall aims of collaborative education are to improve patient safety, promote population health, social inclusion, and advance equitable, culturally informed, quality health care. Dr. Cohen Konrad's research and scholarship focuses on children and families, the use of the arts in health education, health perspectives of vulnerable populations, relational learning, and interprofessional education and collaborative care. She is an associate editor for the *Journal of Interprofessional Care* and the *Journal of Family Social Work*. Her own work is widely published in peer-reviewed journals. She travels nationally and internationally to consult with other universities seeking to enhance collaborative learning and present her scholarship and research.

Kris Hall, M.F.A. (*consultant to the planning committee*), is the program manager for the Center for Excellence in Collaborative Education at the University of New England (UNE), working across the university to provide opportunities for students to learn with, from, and about each other. She is also the program manager for the Substance Abuse and Mental Health Services Administration–funded screening, brief intervention, and referral to treatment (SBIRT) grant awarded to UNE to provide training and education in screening, brief intervention, and referral for treatment for substance use disorders to students, faculty, and community partners from eight health professions. She formerly served as the associate director for Add Verb Productions, promoting performances aimed at bystander intervention in the realms of domestic violence and sexual assault, and eating disorders respectively. As part of a faculty team, she has given national and international presentations and published, on the Interprofessional Team Immersion, a unique curricular resource that was designed in response to student requests for small, interactive, cross-professional learning experiences. Ms.

Hall is a graduate of the Maine College of Art and a past participant at the Skowhegan School of Painting and Sculpture.

Karen Pardue, Ph.D., M.S., RN, CNE, ANEF (*consultant to the planning committee*), is the dean for the Westbrook College of Health Professions. She brings to this role 7 years of experience as the associate dean for academic affairs, providing leadership in health profession curriculum development and outcomes assessment, faculty development, and specialty accreditation expertise. Her research and scholarship focuses on interprofessional (IPE) curriculum development and evaluation. Dr. Pardue led the design and implementation of the University of New England's (UNE's) innovative undergraduate IPE coursework. Her experience in nursing education is diverse, having held faculty and administrative positions in associate, RN to BSN, generic BSN, and master's-level programs. For 10 years, she executed international teaching and leadership roles through a unique RN to BSN partnership program between UNE and Israel College in Tel Aviv, Israel. She is active in statewide and national organizations addressing higher education and the preparation of health professionals. She is an invited member to the National League for Nursing (NLN) Strategic Action Group on Disseminating IPE and Collaborative Practices and led the NLN Task Group on Innovation in Nursing Education. She was appointed by the governor of Maine to the New England Board of Higher Education where she currently chairs the Maine delegation, and she has served as a mentor in the national NLN/Johnson & Johnson Faculty Mentoring program. Dr. Pardue has published and presented widely on innovative pedagogies, IPE, and evidence-based approaches to teaching and learning. She is on the editorial board of *Nurse Educator* and she provides manuscript review for a number of nursing and IPE journals. Dr. Pardue was inducted as a fellow into the Academy of Nursing Education in 2007 and she currently chairs the Fellow Selection Committee. She is a recipient of grant awards from the Arthur Vining Davis Foundations, the Bingham Program Foundation, and a Josiah Macy President's Award targeting IPE curriculum and faculty development.

Roderic I. Pettigrew, Ph.D., M.D., serves as the chief executive officer of engineering health (EnHealth) and is the executive dean for the engineering medicine (EnMed) program at Texas A&M University, in partnership with Houston Methodist Hospital. Dr. Pettigrew also holds the endowed Robert A. Welch Chair in Chemistry. EnHealth is the nation's first comprehensive educational program to fully integrate engineering into all health-related disciplines. EnMed is the nation's first 4-year, fully integrated engineering and medical education curriculum leading to both an M.D. and a master's degree in engineering. An internationally recognized leader in biomedical imaging and bioengineering, Dr. Pettigrew served as the first director for the National Institute of Biomedical Imaging and Bioengineering at the National Institutes of Health (NIH). Prior to his appointment at NIH, he joined the Emory University School of Medicine as a professor of radiology and the Georgia Institute of Technology as a professor of bioengineering. Dr. Pettigrew is well known for pioneering four-dimensional imaging of the cardiovascular system using magnetic resonance imaging. In addition to his numerous achievements, he is an elected member to both the National Academy of Medicine and the National Academy of Engineering. After receiving his B.S. in physics from Morehouse College as a Merrill Scholar, Dr. Pettigrew attended Rensselaer Polytechnic Institute, where he earned his M.S. in nuclear science and engineering. Dr. Pettigrew received his Ph.D. in radiation physics at the Massachusetts Institute of Technology and attained his medical doctorate from Leonard M. Miller School of Medicine at the University of Miami.

Norma Iris Poll-Hunter, Ph.D., is the senior director of human capital initiatives within Diversity Policy and Programs at the Association of American Medical Colleges (AAMC). In this role, she leads a portfolio of career development programs with a focus on diversity and inclusion across the medical education continuum. She serves as the deputy director for the Summer Health Professions Education Program, a national pipeline program to increase diversity in the health professions. She also leads initiatives focused on cultural competence in medical education, building collaborations and partnerships to advance diversity, and research and evaluation projects focused on diversity in the health care workforce. Prior to AAMC, Dr. Poll-Hunter practiced as a bilingual psychologist at a regional hospital in upstate New York. Following receipt of her B.A. from Lehman College, City University of New York, Dr. Poll-Hunter earned her Ph.D. in counseling psychology at the University of Albany, State University of New York.

John-Paul Sánchez, M.D., M.P.H., serves as the president of the Building the Next Generation of Academic Physicians, Inc. (BNGAP), whose mission is to help diverse medical students and residents become aware of academic medicine as a career option and to provide them with the resources to further explore and potentially embark on an academic medicine career. In 2014, he joined the Rutgers New Jersey Medical School as the assistant dean for diversity and inclusion. Dr. Sánchez recently completed terms on the National Hispanic Medical Association and the Hispanic Serving Health Professions Schools and was elected to serve as the co-executive director of Latino Medical Student Association National, a 501(c)(3) nonprofit organization founded to represent, support, educate, and unify U.S. Latino(a) premedical and medical students. He also currently sits on the board of the Callen Lorde LGBT Community Health Center in New York

City. He received his M.D. from Einstein, completed his residency training at Jacobi/Montefiore, and is board certified in emergency medicine. He also holds an M.P.H., with a concentration in the epidemiology of infectious diseases, from the Yale School of Public Health. He is of Puerto Rican ancestry, gay-identified, and was raised in the Bronx, New York City.

Lawrence Sherman, FACEHP, CHCP, is the principal at Meducate Global, LLC, a U.S.-based organization involved in the assessment of global health care education systems worldwide, faculty development for educators of health care professionals, and support of continuing professional development in health care worldwide. He also holds an international development position with the Association for Medical Education in Europe. Mr. Sherman has been involved in medical and interprofessional education, with a concentration in continuing education, for more than 25 years, and has authored numerous scholarly publications and delivered hundreds of presentations worldwide on topics related to medical education. Mr. Sherman is active in the continuing education profession worldwide, with key involvement and participation in organizations, societies, and academic institutions globally. Some of the organizations include the Asia Pacific Medical Education Conference and the Alliance for Continuing Education in the Health Professions. Mr. Sherman is the social media editor for the *Journal for Continuing Education in the Health Professions* and is a reviewer for the *Journal of European CME*, *Medical Teacher*, and the *Asia Pacific Scholar*. Mr. Sherman is a frequent speaker at global health care conferences; examples of his presentations include talks at TEDxMaastricht (http://www.youtube.com/watch?v=YpSd5u_di9w), Singularity University (http://www.youtube.com/watch?v=B4Qkbw8969w), and Villanova University (https://reachmd.com/programs/villanova_health_summit/observations-medical-educator-turned-patient/8078). Frequent lecture topics include faculty training, optimizing presentation and communications skills, interprofessional continuing education, globalizing medical education, humor in medical education, needs assessments and outcomes in health care education, customer service in medicine, understanding learners in medical education, health care communications, and the future of health care education. He often moderates consensus panels and curriculum development meetings and also leads the podium skills training sessions and faculty development workshops. He has also hosted an Internet radio show focusing on key topics in medical education that is broadcast on the ReachMD platform. Mr. Sherman has also been an educator in emergency medicine for the Emergency Medical Institute and the Center for Learning and Innovation of the Northwell Health System in Long Island, New York, and he has lectured in the Healthcare Communications program at the Center for Communicating Science at Stony Brook University, also in New York.

Aliki Thomas, Ph.D., OT (*consultant to the planning committee*), is an associate professor in the School of Physical and Occupational Therapy and an associate member of the Institute of Health Sciences Education, Faculty of Medicine, McGill University. She earned a doctorate in educational psychology with a major in instructional psychology and a minor in applied cognitive science. She completed postdoctoral training at McMaster University in knowledge translation for evidence-based practice. Dr. Thomas's research is guided by the principles of the Scholarship of Practice whereby research, education, and practice are interwoven and interconnected with the aim of improving the health, function, and participation of individuals in our society. Informed by theories from educational psychology, applied cognitive science, and implementation science, and using mixed methodological approaches, Dr. Thomas's research program seeks to understand the developmental trajectory from the classroom, where entry-level evidence-based practice competencies are initially acquired, to the real life "messy" clinical practice context where graduates are expected to navigate multiple influences to provide evidence-based and patient-centered care. Her research program is organized under three main themes: (1) education for evidence-based practices in the health professions, (2) knowledge translation for evidence-based education and clinical practice, and (3) the education–practice nexus. Dr. Thomas has a thriving research lab with several graduate students and postdoctoral fellows. More information about her and her students' research activities can be obtained at https://www.mcgill.ca/keep-lab.

Valerie N. Williams, Ph.D., M.P.A., is a University of Oklahoma Presidential Professor in the Health Sciences Center Graduate College and holds academic appointments in the Colleges of Medicine and Public Health. She serves as the vice provost for academic affairs and faculty development at the University of Oklahoma Health Sciences Center (OUHSC). In this role she has responsibility for campus-wide academic affairs, academic integrity, and faculty development issues. Dr. Williams created the OUHSC Faculty Leadership Program for interprofessional faculty development and mentoring in 1990. During her career she has served as a mentor or coach for more than 1,000 faculty. Dr. Williams founded and directs the federally designated University Center for Excellence in Developmental Disabilities for Oklahoma. She is the senior director for the professional development core of the National Institutes of Health–supported Oklahoma Shared Clinical and Translational Resources Center. Nationally, Dr. Williams serves on the Educational Advisory Committee for the Association of American Medical Colleges (AAMC) Minority Faculty Leadership Development Programs, and she serves as the co-chair (with Dr. Robert Alpern) for the AAMC Physician-Scientist Advisory Panel. Dr. Williams earned a B.S. from

Syracuse University (SU) in biology and psychology (major: genetics), an M.P.A. from the Maxwell School of Citizenship & Public Affairs at SU, and a Ph.D. in allied health sciences from the University of Oklahoma. She is a lifetime member of the Alpha Phi Omega national service organization. She has received several national awards including the AAMC Group on Faculty Affairs Carole J. Bland Phronesis Award honoring "members of the faculty affairs community who exemplify the spirit of phronesis through dedicated and selfless promotion of faculty vitality."

Appendix D

Best Andragogical Practices for Online Learning and Faculty Development

Engage the Audience

- Talk directly to the audience.
- Use the chat function to engage participants in brief conversations.
- Employ a variety of media like videos and Zoom polls.
- Have speakers (or the moderator) talk to each other as though they are having a conversation.
- Ask someone to monitor the chat discussion and have the moderator call on that person to tell the group what is being discussed or questions being asked.
- Project colorful and engaging slides (not overly filled with written text).
- Keep presentations short (less than 10 minutes) and discussions long.
- Ask the audience what they want to get from the session, and gear the conversation in that direction.
- Hire actors to play roles for training faculty on how to run case studies.
- Recognize that audience members may have a deeper understanding of the literature than the speaker.

Be Careful...

- Not to distract participants from the speakers while using the chat function for supplemental discussions.

- When using technologies that take up bandwidth and can slow the transmission of messages (i.e., videos and slide transitions).
- To schedule meetings at times that work for the speakers based on the time zone they are presenting from.
- To avoid excess lighting behind the speaker.

Prepare the Speakers

- Provide an annotated agenda that has the times of when each speaker will talk.
- Test the technology (i.e., share screen) 30 minutes prior to the session.
- Click through all of the slides with the speakers before the session begins.
- Have a backup plan if a speaker's technology fails—move to the next speaker or have someone take over until the speaker returns.
- Remind speakers to turn on/off their videos and mute/unmute their computers at the appropriate times.
- Agree on a system of time keeping.
- Use a waiting room to admit participants and remove disruptive attendees.
- Share cell phone numbers of presenters prior to the session.

SOURCE: Input from individual members of the workshop planning committee (see p. v).

Appendix E

Forum-Sponsored Products

GLOBAL FORUM ON INNOVATION IN HEALTH PROFESSIONAL EDUCATION SUMMARIES AND PROCEEDINGS

nationalacademies.org/ihpeglobalforum

Interprofessional Education for Collaboration: Learning How to Improve Health from Interprofessional Models Across the Continuum of Education to Practice: Workshop Summary (2013)

Establishing Transdisciplinary Professionalism for Improving Health Outcomes: Workshop Summary (2013)

Assessing Health Professional Education: Workshop Summary (2013)

Building Health Workforce Capacity Through Community-Based Health Professional Education: Workshop Summary (2014)

Empowering Women and Strengthening Health Systems and Services Through Investing in Nursing and Midwifery Enterprise: Lessons from Lower-Income Countries: Workshop Summary (2015)

Measuring the Impact of Interprofessional Education on Collaborative Practice and Patient Outcomes (2015)

Envisioning the Future of Health Professional Education: Workshop Summary (2015)

A Framework for Educating Health Professionals to Address the Social Determinants of Health (2016)

Exploring the Role of Accreditation in Enhancing Quality and Innovation in Health Professions Education: Proceedings of a Workshop (2016)

Future Financial Economics of Health Professional Education: Proceedings of a Workshop (2017)

Exploring a Business Case for High-Value Continuing Professional Development: Proceedings of a Workshop (2018)

Improving Health Professional Education and Practice Through Technology: Proceedings of a Workshop (2018)

A Design Thinking, Systems Approach to Well-Being Within Education and Practice: Proceedings of a Workshop (2019)

Strengthening the Connection Between Health Professions Education and Practice: Proceedings of a Joint Workshop (2019)

The Role of Nonpharmacological Approaches to Pain Management: Proceedings of a Workshop (2019)

Educating Health Professionals to Address the Social Determinants of Mental Health (2020)

NATIONAL ACADEMY OF MEDICINE PERSPECTIVE PAPERS

Breaking the Culture of Silence on Physician Suicide (2016)

I Felt Alone But I Wasn't: Depression Is Rampant Among Doctors in Training (2016)

Defining Community-Engaged Health Professional Education: A Step Toward Building the Evidence (2017)

100 Days of Rain: A Reflection on the Limits of Physician Resilience (2017)

A Multifaceted Systems Approach to Addressing Stress Within Health Professions Education and Beyond (2017)

Addressing Burnout, Depression, and Suicidal Ideation in the Osteopathic Profession: An Approach That Spans the Physician Life Cycle (2017)

Burnout, Stress, and Compassion Fatigue in Occupational Therapy Practice and Education: A Call for Mindful, Self-Care Protocols (2017)

Promoting Well-Being in Psychology Graduate Students at the Individual and Systems Levels (2017)

Stress-Induced Eating Behaviors of Health Professionals: A Registered Dietitian Nutritionist Perspective (2017)

Breaking Silence, Breaking Stigma (2017)

Breaking the Culture of Silence: The Role of State Medical Boards (2017)

The Role of Accreditation in Achieving the Quadruple Aim (2017)

Nursing, Trauma, and Reflective Writing (2018)

The Role of Health Care Profession Accreditors in Promoting Health and Well-Being Across the Learning Continuum (2018)

Utilizing a Systems and Design Thinking Approach for Improving Well-Being Within Health Professions' Education and Health Care (2019)

Compassionate, Patient-Centered Care in the Digital Age (2019)

What Is the Value of Social Determinants of Health in Dental Education? (2020)

Health Professional Education Student Volunteerism Amid COVID-19: How a Diverse, Interprofessional Team of Health Students Created a Volunteer Model to Support Essential Workers (2020)

Educating Health Professions Educators to Address the "isms" (2020)

Learning from the Global Response to the COVID-19 Pandemic: An Interprofessional Perspective on Health Professions Education (2020)